Dear Alicia,

This is a small gift to
thank you for
your card.

Best wishes

Alex Bel
11/10/09.

FABULOUSLY BEAUTIFUL YOU!

Prof. Dr. Paul Ling Tai

&

Dr. Alex DeSouza

Optimal Health

Institute

Health Secrets USA

In conjunction with

United Writers Press, Inc.

P.O. Box 326

Tucker, Georgia USA 30085-0326

Copyright 2009 Prof. Dr. Paul Ling Tai

&

Dr. Alex DeSouza

ISBN- 13:978-1-934216-92-7

Printed in the USA

Disclaimer

This publication is designed to provide scientific, authoritative and personal anecdotal information in regard to the subject matter covered. The reader understands that the authors and publisher are not engaged in rendering professional services.

If you require medical, psychological or any other expert assistance, please seek the services of a professional.

The information, personal experiences, anecdotal stories, procedures and suggestions contained within this book are not intended to replace the services of a trained health care professional or to serve as a replacement for a professional medical doctor's advice and care. You should consult a health care professional regarding any of the information, ideas, personal experiences, anecdotal stories, procedures, supplements, drug therapies or any other information from this book.

The author and publisher hereby specifically disclaim any and all liability arising directly or indirectly from the use or application of any of the products, ideas, procedures, drug therapies, or suggestions contained in this book and any errors, omissions, and inaccuracies in the information contained herein.

The treatments and supplements included in this book are for identification purposes only and are not intended to recommend or endorse the product.

Important Warning

This book is intended for readers and physicians to evaluate hormone deficiencies occurring in the human body; however, it is not intended for pregnant or nursing women, nor is it intended for children below the age of 18.

Optimal and deficient values presented within this book do not necessarily correspond to the reference values found in local laboratories. The values and references used in this book are purely subjective and come from the author's own personal experiences and by other physicians who have shared their experiences.

The reader should not base his or her assessment solely on the values given in this book. Hormonal imbalances are determined by laboratories, and corrective approaches are determined by a trained medical professional.

Laboratory values within this book constitute only some of the information the reader should gather. Much more emphasis should be placed on clinical evaluation, signs, and symptoms. Many other clinical and laboratory tests should be used before deciding on a diagnosis and/ or treatment. A reader should always seek a physician's advice before deciding to institute any form of medical treatment.

CONTENTS

Section I

Section 2

ACKNOWLEDGMENTS

My sincere & profound thanks for my partner, Dr. Alex DeSouza. Special thanks to Katherine M. Lee for all her encouragement & help. Also, thanks to Lisa Klink for her help with the book.

Victor Solaris, Ada & Arlene Tai for the beautiful book cover & hours of work. Thank You!

Prof. Dr. Paul Ling Tai

My sincere gratitude and love to my patients, and to my family, a doctor without its patients is not a complete doctor and a man without his family is not a complete man!

Dr. Alex DeSouza

FOREWORD

A NEW VIEW OF AGING

Gradually, our perception of what it means to grow old is changing. The old concept of what it meant to be old typically involved things like wrinkles, Alzheimer's disease, bone loss, and muscle loss, and that is why people did not want to get old. Today, we are more concerned about our functional biologic aging than our chronologic age. For example, Sophia Loren, who just turned 74, recently posed for a calendar wearing nothing but a pair of earrings. She looked nothing like the old concept of what an old person looks like. The world has changed dramatically & permanently.

Men and women are now doing things in their senior years that they would never dreamt of being able to do in their twenties. Today, the capabilities of human potential have gone far beyond what we could have imagined just several decades ago.

This book will change your perception of *Aging*, and the impact to your health and the health of your patients from the new technologies of *Anti-Aging Medicine*.

Anyone can find disease. What sets us apart is that we look for health. Our objective is to find health and enhance it so that we can make it possible for the massive baby boomer population to do the things that they really want to do. We have to start thinking out of the box.

In 1997, *the American Academy of Anti-Aging Medicine* was started by 12 founders; today at 2009, *A4M/ WAAAM World -American Academy of Anti-Aging Medicine* have over 100,000 doctors participating in our worldwide Anti-Aging Medical conferences, representing over 105 countries. There are over 500,000 subscribers to A4M/WAAAM Anti-Aging Medical News.

Dr. Paul Ling Tai and Dr. Alex DeSouza are teachers and leaders in the field of Anti-Aging Medicine & Plastic Surgery Regenerative Medicine, teaching us that beauty, from the "inside out", consists not only of looking beautiful, but feeling beautiful & healthy! This book represents the latest medical technology in the pursuit of: *Looking younger, Feeling stronger and Living longer.*

Dr. Robert M. Goldman, MD., DO., PhD. FAASP.
Chairman, A4M/WAAM
Founder, Nat. Acad. Sports Med.
Chairman, Int. Med. Commission
Chairman, Jr. Olympics Med. Com
Sp. Adv. Pres. Com. Phys. Fit. & Sp
W. Chairman, IFBB Med. Com

Chapter 1

Searching for beauty and finding health

"To keep the body in good health is a duty... otherwise we shall not be able to keep our mind strong and clear."

~Buddha

Perhaps one of the most magical things about life is that we never know where life is going to take us. When I was growing up in the countryside of Brazil, it wasn't very clear to me what I wanted to be when I grew up. What was clear to me, however, was that I had a strong fondness for sports and I was extremely curious — almost to the point that one could consider me to be a mini scientist. Even before I started school, I was a very inquisitive young boy.

As a young child growing up in the 1960s, television shows such as Time Tunnel, Star Trek, and Dr. Kildare had a profound impact on my life. Dr. Kildare — a NBC medical drama television series -- was perhaps the reason I always wanted to become a doctor and move from Brazil to the United States. I found myself captivated watching Kildare, a young intern in a large metropolitan hospital trying to learn his profession, dealing with problems of the patients while winning the respect of the senior doctor. It wasn't that Brazil didn't have good medicine; it's just that the United States seemed to have a special magic about it that combined well-organized systems, high technology, and the desire to move forward in science.

> **Did You Know?**
>
> The United States and Brazil perform the highest number of plastic surgery procedures in the world each year.

The 1960s was not only a time for great television shows; it was also a significant turning point for general medicine, plastic surgery, wellness, and anti-aging. Facelifts became a reality in the 1960s as well as cosmetic procedures such as Botox®. In the era of John F. Kennedy when Americans believed that universe was the limit, sophisticated methods for maintaining health such as birth control pills, large-scale vaccinations, and ICUs were implemented.

No matter how you plan or how you try to see the future, when the ball starts to roll, it's hard to tell where the ball is going to stop.

From Sports to Medical School

I started practicing soccer, Judo, and various water sports as a young child. While playing soccer, I learned early on about the team mentality — that nobody wins without the team. With Judo, I learned that persistence and discipline is crucial for the way that we conduct our lives.

As I look back now and see my own kids growing up in America, it's fascinating to see what made me make the turns that I did in my life. Being a country boy from Brazil, I could never imagine myself practicing medicine in the United States.

I truly believe that my experiences in sports as well as my natural scientific curiosity moved me through high school and into medicine. Not only did I strive for good grades throughout high school; while attending college in Brazil, I passed the required medical school entrance exam with ease.

> "Health is a state of complete harmony of the body, mind and spirit. When one is free from physical disabilities and mental distractions, the gates of the soul open."
>
> ~B.K.S. Iyeng

It was in my third year of medical school during rotations that I fell in love with plastic surgery. I will never forget seeing how doctors were able to miraculously transform the appearance of a young girl who had been severely burned. I was fascinated with how plastic surgery could change people's lives in such broad ways. The diversification of plastic surgery simply amazed me. Plastic surgery came to me as one of the few medical fields that offered an array of opportunities to treat children, the elderly, men, and women. What other medical fields could allow me to treat cancer patients, burn victims, and also give patients back their youth and beauty?

Continuing the Search

Science has always been a major part of my life — especially in medical school where I took on a variety of projects. I started a medical magazine for medical students in Brazil. It was the first time that Brazilian medical students produced a medical journal. In addition, I combined my love of science with my love for the written word and published several papers as well as a few books including one about manipulating the taboos in our life. My curiosity about life, nutrition, and beauty prompted me to write a book about the liver in which I approached several theories about the physiology of a hangover and skin lesions (or liver spots). The combination of these experiences allowed me to develop a stronger me where beauty and health were together.

Positive Influences

It's absolutely amazing what kind of influence not only good people, but also bad people, can have in your life. As a parent, we constantly strive to have good people surround our children so that they are shielded, yet allowed to build their dreams which can be bigger than themselves. As a physician, I think we should have the same responsibilities as to who we associate with.

Because I had an obsession to be the best possible plastic surgeon, I decided to move to America to continue my search for health and beauty as well as further my medical training. I was already a full, board-certified, well-established plastic surgeon in Brazil when I participated in a fellowship at the University of Alabama in Birmingham. Among the many brilliant plastic surgeons that were my role models and mentors were Dr. Louis Vasconez and Dr. Psillakis. They instilled in me an excitement and incredible enthusiasm for developing noninvasive procedures that are more comfortable for the patient, has minimal down time, are less traumatic, and are more affordable for the average person.

I can never thank enough all the professors and others that I've trained with including the ones in Brazil. As much as I'd like to create a list of those to thank, I won't because there are so many people and I don't want to miss any of them. While some of these people were in my life for only a short period of time, others have remained in my life for years.

My Search for Beauty

"Just because you're not sick doesn't mean you're healthy."

~Author Unknown

For the last 25 years, I've been looking for a way to produce a more youthful and beautiful appearance with the least amount of disruption to the patient's lifestyle. To my surprise, I learned that the very same procedure could be successfully performed on two different patients, but yield two different results. I asked myself, "Why is it that some patients do not respond the same way? Why are one patient's results far more superior to that of another patient? And why are some patients not as satisfied even though the technique is homogeneous?" I started to learn that you cannot be pretty if you are not healthy. I was surprised to find that beauty actually lies within health. What surprised me even more was learning why beauty has been separated from health since they are really one in the same thing.

Everywhere you look in nature, beauty and health are together. For example, a pretty tree is a healthy tree; a pretty animal is a healthy animal; and pretty water is healthy water. There is definitely an intrinsic relationship between beauty and health throughout nature that cannot be separated. Unfortunately, in our case, beauty and health has been separated thanks to the media and the cosmetic industry. This is why there is such a gap between results and satisfaction of plastic surgery procedures. If the physician does not approach beauty and health at the same time while treating a patient, good results will not be obtained.

The Biggest Question

> "Without health, there is no point to anything."
>
> ~Everett Mámor

The biggest question that many people ask today is, "Is it possible to have a facelift without surgery? Is it possible to get your youth back and look pretty without surgery?" It's no secret that people want to look good. After all, it's a very competitive world out there. Looking good is not just the desire of Americans; it's a global mentality. Everyone wants to look as young and good as possible. Of course the media doesn't help matters much by continuing to display unrealistic situations where people need to look optimal all the time.

If you were to ask ten people if they'd like to look younger and more attractive, most likely they'd all say yes. However, if you were to ask those same people whether or not they'd like to be put to sleep in order to have a major surgery to look younger and then take four to six weeks to recover, chances are they would say "no!" Most likely it's because they either can't afford to take the time off or they would rather not take such a radical approach just to look good.

But, if you were to ask those same people if they'd like to look younger and more attractive without surgery and without interrupting their normal lifestyle activities by undergoing several small procedures, I bet they'd say "yes!" Until recently however, this would have been a problem because there hadn't been enough procedures or treatments developed that could actually accomplish that.

It's clear that people want a youthful looking face and the classic shape of healthy body. As stated earlier, we now have at our fingertips a variety of noninvasive procedures that can help. In fact, the progress and the speed in which things come out on the market is absolutely amazing. Fortunately, we are now able to do a lot for your appearance and for your health. Procedures like breast surgery, tummy tuck, liposuction, thigh surgery, arm treatment, and skincare for face and body are a tremendous help to accomplish what we are looking for, which is a good and youthful appearance of the body and face.

Beauty around the world

The search for beauty and health is not only the fight of one person or one country. We are starting to see what is called "cosmetic medicine without barriers." When we review what is happening around the world and talk to prominent surgeons, we find that the search for beauty, health, and anti-aging is growing faster than any other specialty. This is the desire of everyone, not just people of one country or one culture. Patients and doctors alike are searching for ways to look younger, feel stronger, and live longer.

The Data Monitor, a research firm based in the United Kingdom, shows that cosmetic surgery is raising. The British will be spending over £1.5 billion pounds by the year 2011. Surprisingly, the rate at which the British are seeking cosmetic procedures is rising faster than that of the United States.

A Piece of History
More noninvasive procedures have been developed in the last four years than in the last 4,000 years of medicine.

This trend to look good isn't limited to just the United States and Great Britain, however. Tremendous growth of cosmetic surgeries are also seen in South America as well as "BRIC" countries, which refers to the new group of developing countries that include Brazil, Russia, India, and China. A huge increase in cosmetic surgeries and noninvasive procedures can even be seen in conservative Middle Eastern countries such as Dubai and Israel.

Beauty By the Numbers

Dr. Renato Saltz, a plastic surgeon from Park City, UT and president-elect of the American Society for Aesthetic Plastic Surgery, says that the cosmetic surgery industry is rapidly growing around the world. Dr. Goes, of Brazil, estimates the cosmetic medicine industry to be increasing by 12 to 18 percent annually.

There were nearly 11.7 million surgical and non-surgical cosmetic procedures performed in the United States in 2007, as reported by the American Society for Aesthetic Plastic Surgery (ASAPS). Out of those, non-surgical procedures accounted for 82% of the total!!!

It's clear to me that people are looking for and will continue to seek out noninvasive methods in order to look good, feel good, and live longer. Furthermore, because cosmetic procedures are much more affordable for everyone, there is no question that this trend is not just a desire of the rich and famous.

What's ahead?

While it's possible to perform a facelift without surgery, is it possible to perform a facelift without surgery without any regards to anti-aging or to treating your health? The answer to this is a big, fat, NO! Without wellness, without hormone balance, without a proper diet, no amount of plastic surgery or money will make you look good if you are not healthy.

Today we know that only when noninvasive procedures are combined with wellness and anti-aging, optimal health can be achieved. Throughout this book, you'll be able to learn not only what can be done today, but how history has made these innovations possible. We talk about how the facelift has transformed itself over the years. We tell you how you can repair your damaged skin, therefore giving you the appearance of youth. And the cosmetic procedures and anti-aging care discussed in this book refer not to just your face, but to the entire body.

After all, your face is only ten percent of your body and your body ages the same way that your face does.

An Innovative Approach to Health and Beauty

Together with the knowledge and friendship of Dr. Paul Tai, we've developed a breakthrough program in medicine-- one that addresses three important parts of health — beauty, wellness, and anti-aging. I hope that Dr. Tai and I will be able to help you as much as we've helped our patients and ourselves, for that matter.

We will reveal how diet, nutrition, hormone balance, hydration, brain health, and exercise all play a part in maximizing your beauty.

All recommendations that I make in this book I've experienced directly or through my patients, family, and friends. Therefore, please take home these valuable lessons that can help you maintain your health, and give you back your youth and beauty. The goal for all of us is to look younger, feel stronger, and live longer.

I hope you will enjoy the journey through this book. You will get a snapshot of the past, you will see the energy of the present, and you will get a taste of what the future has in store for us.

Chapter 2

The "Lux" Paradigm

"Advertisers in general bear a large part of the responsibility for the deep feelings of inadequacy that drive women to psychiatrists, pills, or the bottle."

~Marya Mannes, *But Will It Sell?*, 1964

In order to realize that you cannot have true beauty without good health, it's helpful to travel back through history to see just how health and beauty became separated in the first place.

So the story begins...

Unknowingly, the quest for beauty started very early one grayish, chilly autumn morning in Jamestown, the new Colony of Virginia, when a new type of professional arriving from England in the second ship began work. Taking advantage of the animal butchering activities that were occurring at the homesteads and farms, these "new professionals" collected the animal fat. In the spring, they combined the excess fat melted from the animal sacrifice with ashes. They used ashes from the winter fires and mixed them with discarded cooking grease that had accumulated throughout the year to create, in chemical terms: sodium, potassium, salt and fat acids – or in layman's terms, soap. Surrounded by mystery, these new professionals developed a product that revolutionized the way that people cleansed themselves and their household possessions. This new breed of craftsman became known as "soap makers."

Several of the passengers who arrived at Jamestown on the second ship from England were soap makers. High taxes and stories of corruption surround the initial consumption of this almost magical product. The business was so prosperous that in 1622, King James I granted a monopoly to a soap maker for $100,000 a year. The heavily taxed luxury item was much in demand. Soap was used by the rich and famous for personal hygiene as well as by physicians in their treatment of diseases of the skin. It made people's living conditions healthier.

And even earlier.......

While it is almost impossible to track the historical beginnings of soap, traces of soap-like material were found as early as 3000 B.C. in Babylon, known today as Iraq. It's also very likely the Egyptians knew and used this kind of product to treat diseases; therefore, its main function was for health purposes. Personal hygiene levels seemed to have peaked during the time of the Roman Empire, which was known for its famous luxurious baths.

It is likely that the Romans also contributed to the word "soap". The word has been said to come from a mountain in Ancient Rome where animals were sacrificed. At the famous mountain named Mt. Sapo, a phenomenon occurred every time it rained. Rainwater washed out the mixed, melted fat from the dead animals. The melted fat then combined with wood ashes from the sacrifice rituals and the clay soil along the Tiber River to produce a mixture that would make the stones at the base of the mountain much cleaner than the stones of surrounding areas. Soon the local women from the Mt. Sapo area discovered that this mixture could be very helpful with their daily activities of washing clothes and their household possessions. The term 'soap' then became a household word.

The Middle Ages was a dark period of history and was a dark time for soap as well. After the fall of the Roman Empire in 476 AD, hygiene habits throughout all of Europe drastically declined. The lack of personal hygiene habits included less frequent bathing which was directly related to the development of great plagues in the Middle Ages--particularly the Black Death that struck in the 14th century.

The soap renaissance

In the 17th century, the rebirth of soap paved the way for improved living conditions and newly developed lifestyle habits, particularly in Europe and England, where soap was used for washing clothes and home objects as well as for personal hygiene. Interestingly enough though, personal bathing was not a frequent activity among the nobles of Europe. Queen Elizabeth was often criticized for her uncommon frequency of bathing. In the eyes of the British noble family, she was taking too many baths (perhaps four baths a year).

> **Did you know?**
>
> Taking a bath four times a year was considered to be abnormal by British nobles in the 17th century.

The soap industry, which was already a significant source of income for the noble families in England, also became an important source of income for the habitants of the new colonies, particularly the new Colony of Virginia. A review of Captain John Smith's records revealed that the exportation of ashes (an important ingredient in soap) to Europe earned over $1 million per year. Even with all the success of soap, at this time it was still primarily used for cleaning and washing clothes rather than for personal hygiene.

From hygiene to beauty

As odd as it may seem, there is something very special about the historic story of soap because it really explains the important transition that was made between health and hygiene to beauty and wellness. In the early 1900s, many of the landmarks of modern medicine such as surgery and anesthesia remained experimental and simply were not available to the common person. The best we could hope for at that time was good hygiene. Then all of a sudden, one of the most important products used for hygiene — soap — was also marketed for cosmetic purposes.

When you look back through history, no other product has made the kind of impact on medicine, marketing and the cosmetic industry like soap has. Not even sophisticated machines such as lasers, CT scans, MRIs can compete with soap. If you look around in a hospital, nothing makes as big of a difference as soap does.

By sensing its potential and realizing how extremely simple and accessible soap is, the industry created an entire soap empire that focused on marketing to the beauty industry. Appealing to the consumer's desire to look good didn't start until soap underwent the transformation from hygiene to beauty. There's no question in my mind that the soap movement is what lead us to where we are today in terms of cosmetic medicine.

The increasing popularity of soap

In the late 1800s, Andrew Pears was the first to establish a subtle relationship between soap and beauty. Pears realized that the common folk who worked outside had tanned faces and needed a soap that was gentler on their skin. He developed a method for removing the impurities from the soap.

During the 19th century, a very important milestone in soap history was reached in America when French chemist, Nicholas Leblanc, patented the process of making soap using mainly raw material. Because soap making then became a large-scale operation, it became affordable for the regular population. This scientific discovery allowed soap making to become the fastest growing industry by the middle 1800's.

Once again, despite the immense success of the soap industry, soap was still being used more for cleaning and washing clothes than for personal hygiene or facial rejuvenation. However, in 1899 something happened. The Lever Brothers developed a popular product known as Sunshine Flakes. In the 1900's, Sunshine Flakes, which was intended for cleaning at home, was also being used by women for personal hygiene.

With the success of the Sunshine Flakes, the Lever Company decided to change the product's name to Lux. They believed that Lux was a catchier name and sounded more luxurious — perfect for marketing it toward personal hygiene and facial care. More important than the actual product, the creation of Lux marked the beginning of a very important battle between aggressive marketing campaigns and the science itself.

Marketing strategies vs. science

Unfortunately, history has shown that effective marketing strategies are far more powerful in capturing the public's interest than any scientific study. In the 1940s, the Lever Brothers Corporation decided to contract famous movie stars such as Judy Garland and Betty Davis to appear in their Lux advertisements. This new marketing strategy of using famous movie stars to represent beauty products was so effective that it still remains a powerful marketing tool today. The Lever Brothers campaign continued on using the classic slogan "Nine or ten movie stars use Lux". Almost sixty years later, despite all of the scientific progress, this powerful slogan still lives and remains a tremendous marketing tool.

The 20th century became a mark in the history of health care and facial rejuvenation. The Lux history sent a strong message to the powerful cosmetic and pharmaceutical industries, which have become a mega enterprise today. On the birth of the 21st century this business model remains useful in the cosmetics and beauty products markets.

The real deal on soap

Although Lux has had six decades of enormous success, I would be shocked if even one out of 50 movie stars were actually using Lux soap on their faces for beauty purposes. In fact, it doesn't matter what type of soap one uses. The truth is — soap is a detergent-- a mixture of vegetable or animal fat with the alkali produced derivative of fat known as fat acids. The fat acid has a powerful detergent action, which allows the fat to be mixed and finally removed. While this property is tremendously effective for cleaning household surfaces, it is not at all suitable for cleaning faces.

Because there was a shortage of fat during World War I, the industry was forced to search for chemical alternatives and to discover new methods of cleaning. This led to a great advance on the production of synthetic soaps and detergents. However, even the high-tech products of today can damage the structure and function of our normal skin. The more we understand about the skin structure, the more we believe that soaps and detergents should not be used on the face under in any circumstance.

> "Advertising may be described as the science of arresting the human intelligence long enough to get money from it." ~Stephen Butler Leacock, quoted in Michael Jackman, *Crown's Book of Political Quotations*, 1982

Conventional soaps are very caustic and can remove the natural protection of the skin's surface. Due to chemical differences between the skin and the soap, the product can cause allergic reactions and chemical burns that in time will damage the skin.

If you need to remove make-up, environmental residues, or excess oils, use a skin cleanser that contains no soap or detergent in the formula, which will be less toxic to your skin. There are several good products on the market for cleansing of the skin. Because no soaps and detergents are in these formulas, they do not cause skin damage.

Of course, strong market campaigns are still pushing soap products and Lux remains firm on the course. If you go to the supermarket, you will see several soaps that claim to help keep your skin young and beautiful; however, it is a fact that conventional soap will do your face much more harm than good and I'm quite sure you won't find any movie stars using it.

The Lux Paradigm

We enter the 21st century with what we call the Lux Paradigm, which is where our dreams are becoming realities. What we ask for, we now have. The Lux Paradigm is the possibility of today. You'll be able to repair your skin and make a difference in your looks. Being able to intervene to control your health and your looks has gone from becoming a dream to becoming a reality. Through a series of noninvasive procedures, people are literally able to change their lives.

The Lux Paradigm has shifted the belief that health and beauty cannot be changed to the belief that while aging is inevitable, aging is not and we *can* make a difference. And the difference is there for everybody because it's affordable. This goal is reachable for everybody — not just the rich and famous. Believe it or not, at one time, soap was only for the rich and famous. Just as soap has become available to everyone, so have many other cosmetic products such as noninvasive cosmetic procedures.

Moisturizer is no friend of your skin!!

Another way that health has been separated from beauty is through the cosmetic industry and their misleading advertisements regarding moisturizers. There really is nothing wrong with moisturizers themselves--the problem is that the media usually circulates inaccurate or exaggerated claims about the benefits of the product. Contrary to what advertisements may tell you, there is nothing magical about moisturizers. It is simply not possible to accomplish skin rejuvenation with moisturizer cream alone.

Don't get me wrong; there are good products on the market as long as you know what you are using and for what purpose. But your expectations should be based on reality. As mentioned earlier about soap, you should interpret all advertisements with a considerable amount of criticism and dismiss the concept that moisturizers are superpower products. I hate to burst anyone's bubble, but the truth is, there are no such things as miracle moisturizers that will erase the signs of aging. I'll explain why in just a few minutes.

> **A Piece of History**
>
> In the second century AD, Galen, the chief physician of the Gladiators, invented the first "cold cream" by mixing melted white wax, olive oil, rosebud, and water. Although many modifications were made to the original formula, Galen's cold cream became the centerpiece of the growing billion-dollar market of the 20th century cosmetic and beauty industry.

The origins of moisturizers

Just before the Civil War, Dr. Thereon T. Ponds, modified a second century A.D. cold cream formulation created by Galen, a Greek physician. Pond's product line and company grew into what eventually became known as Ponds® cream in 1961. Ponds' cream became the best-known moisturizer cream ever and since 1976, remains with the same formula. Because it has had a tremendously successful advertising life, it is fair to say that Ponds' cream initiated the modern era of the moisturizer cream although it was originally created for the treatment of dry skin. Unfortunately, the properties of this popular cream have been exaggerated through misleading advertisements that claim it rejuvenates the skin and contains anti-aging properties.

There are no shortcuts!

Smooth and silky, well-hydrated skin does not seem to be related to moisturizers. Two good examples are the skin of children and the condition of the skin after shaving. In the particular case of men, shaving removes old, dead cells from the surface of the skin, and that removal gives the feeling of smooth and silky tissue. In the case of children, they have yet to be exposed to harmful, external factors such as the sun.

More evidence exists that moisturizers damage the skin more than they provide benefits to it. In fact, moisturizers can exacerbate dermatological problems such as acne, rosacea, and seborrhea and clogged pores. For the majority of people, dry skin is a temporary condition most likely due to effects of external factors such as cold, wind, and sunlight. As soon as the cause is removed and the natural process of skin restoration has started, the problem will be corrected.

The skin has a well-known regular cycle that should be respected. The occasional and temporary use of moisturizer cream can be beneficial in those cases. Even in that type of condition, though, moisturizers should be used for only a short period of time. Despite what the packages may say, long-term use of moisturizers does not provide any benefit to the texture, appearance, or health of the skin.

The health problems of skin restoration and skin rejuvenation are a complex process and need to be seen as such. Several surgical procedures and medical treatments are necessary to give the skin the best appearance possible. There are no shortcuts!! Each case should be treated as an independent case. A skin condition cannot be corrected with a simple application of one cream; therefore, moisturizers need to be used with the right expectation and not with false claims.

Moisturizers do more harm than good

The long-term use of moisturizers can produce three significant adverse effects: addiction, sensitivity, and even an acceleration of the aging process. Addiction results from the overuse of the moisturizer, which can give a false sensation of improvement of dryness. The moisturizer over the skin only masks the defect and problems of the skin. As the moisturizer evaporates, the skin again becomes exposed and the defects are even more severe because the moisturizer has not changed anything on the skin's structure itself. The patient that uses moisturizers every day for several days or several times a day cannot tolerate the feeling of dryness and keeps using the moisturizer, which has become a true addiction.

Sensitivity results from the continuous application of the moisturizer cream, which slows down the exfoliation rate of the old skin and, therefore, affects the normal cycle of the skin and impairs the new and health skin formation.

Generally, after using moisturizer cream daily for a few years, patients are presented with dry and very sensitive skin. The sensitive skin is now easily irritated by factors such as wind, cold, makeup, and other facial products. That sensitivity leads to the use of more moisturizer cream, and consequently, a vicious addiction cycle is started that keeps damaging the skin with continued moisturizer use.

Beauty by the Numbers

The topical wrinkle reducing product market generated over $1billion in sales in 2004, and doubled in 2006!!!

The truth about moisturizers

Although there is a widespread belief that moisturizers have a beneficial effect on wrinkles, the truth is that long-term use of moisturizers only leads to addiction that increases skin sensitivity, which ultimately leads to more addiction. Several scientific studies demonstrate that women who are dependent on moisturizers have more sensitive skin, show signs of aging, and have more prominent wrinkles. Their skin is usually thin and dry, irrigated with unhealthy signs of aging, and is intolerant to make-up.

It is a fact that moisturizers used daily can create more problems than benefits. Moisturizers do not increase the amount of water on the skin. Moisturizers do not restore the damaged skin and neither are they able to prevent aging.

Whose fault is it?

It is wrong and almost malicious to say if a woman does not use moisturizers, a woman's youth and beauty will be lost forever. Nowadays, the cosmetic industry has developed and implemented such powerful marketing strategies, that even doctors who specialize in the treatment of the skin often recommend the use of moisturizers. Little do they know that only a continuous and vigorous restoration program can attempt to correct damaged skin cells.

It is important to understand that optimal appearance and health of the skin depends on the perfect function of its cells, associated with local factors such as ideal levels of hormones, adequate nutrients and of course, daily consumption of large amounts of water. You'll notice, there was no mention of moisturizers. It's important to take care of your skin from the inside out, rather than just the outside in. Hence, it is natural for beauty and health to go hand-in-hand.

Where the cosmetic medicine industry is heading is anyone's guess. With the speed that new procedures and treatments are being developed, one can just imagine what is yet to come. Let's not underestimate what is available today. There are a lot of things that can be done today to reach our goal to look good, feel good, and live longer.

As we enjoy the present day, just imagine the possibilities and what a beautiful and bright future we have ahead of us.

⚘ Dr. De Souza'a Beauty Secret ⚘

Soap should never be used on the face on a regular basis. However, in some special situations, your physician may recommend a few exceptions. Our preference nowadays is to use nontoxic products—preferably natural ones that have a chemical structure compatible with the delicate structure of the skin.

The new technology of today allows us to add products such as vitamins, nutrients and antioxidants to the cleansers used for skin hygiene. Not even hot water is recommended for use on the face on a regular basis. This is an attempt to protect the fine and delicate surface of the skin.

Moisturizers alone are not enough. As a matter of fact, chronic use and abuse of moisturizers can damage your skin. Skin needs exfoliation, nutrition, and protection. It's important to note that nutrition comes from inside out, not outside in. It's impossible to have beautiful skin without balanced hormones, nutrition, and adequate hydration.

In its history, soap did have and still has important roles in the promotion of health but definitely not with facial rejuvenation. With its mysterious origins, successes, and promises, soap teaches us an important lesson. You should always look at any marketing campaign for any product with a critical eye. It is important not to forget the common wisdom that teaches us, "If something seems to be too good to be true--it probably is."

☙ Dr. De Souza'a Beauty Secret ❧

It's essential that we learn to manage our health as well as our looks. Doctors are trained to treat disease, but not necessarily how to make you healthy and look good. There is actually a big difference between not having a disease and being healthy. The only way to take responsibility is through knowledge. Therefore, the more you educate yourself about things you can do, the better you'll be able to make yourself healthier, look better, and live longer.

It's up to you to climb into the driver's seat and search for your beauty, while also searching for your health.

Chapter 3

Time is not on your side

"Time may be a great healer, but it's a lousy beautician."

~Author Unknown

Regardless of how healthy you may be, aging is a reality and time will ultimately take a toll on all of us.

The Rolling Stones can make their melody, "Time is on my side", famous but they definitely cannot make it true. As far as life is concerned, time is not on our side. From the moment we are born, the clock is ticking and ticking, and nothing stops the aging process. Everything in the universe ages or changes, and our bodies are no exception.

Attempts to search for the mystical Fountain of Youth date back to as far as 3500 BC. Needless to say, no Fountain of Youth has ever been found and nobody can live forever. Over time, different degenerative conditions occur in every part of our body through a process we know as aging. Although aging is not desirable for many people, it should never be considered a disease.

Breaking records

A Piece of History

In 1900, the life expectancy was approximately fifty years of age, and nowadays, it is closer to eighty years.

Numerous studies have shown that various procedures and lifestyle modifications can make a tremendous difference in how long we live. The US 2000 census report counted 50,454 individuals in the USA alone who were over 100 years of age and more than 450,000 worldwide.

Longer life expectancies broke all age records in the 20th century. After all, for the majority of the 70 million years that we've existed as a species, humans have only survived with a life expectancy of twenty-five years or less (contrary to some Biblical descriptions of people living longer than 900 years). No human remains either in the prehistoric era or in any other era have ever been found to be older than about fifty years of age. Furthermore, no archeological or geological evidence exists indicating that a human body can live beyond 120 to 130 years of age.

New scientific studies have focused on those individuals who live longer to see if there is anything that we can learn from them. More scientific studies may be necessary to understand the process of aging and how we can interfere with the intention of prolonging life.

In an interesting study published in *Scientific America* in June 2002, Professor Olshansky, a professor of public health at the University of Illinois, Chicago, described a statement from fifty-one scientists that studied aging. They issued a warning to the public insisting in Dr. Olshansky's words "that no anti-aging remedy on the market today has been proven effective. Under the light of the current signs, aging cannot be stopped, neither reversed nor slowed on its natural process." A number of scientists are looking at current research and are hoping that one day we will provide methods to slow our inevitable decline. Perhaps we will be able to extend human life even longer; however, that day has not yet dawned.

Living longer

> **Did you know?**
>
> Mrs. Jeanne L. Calment is documented in the Guinness Book of Records as the world's oldest verified person. She died on August 4, 1997 at the age of 122 and 164 days old.

Saturday was a beautiful day in the conference room of the hotel in New Orleans, and the room was packed with doctors eager to learn more about aging and its process. When a professor presented a film showing one of his clients, the conference crowd of important physicians fell into a deep silence. The short clip was a wakeup call for each person in the room because immediately a series of questions emerged in the minds of all.

It was very exciting to see the fragile, docile and friendly woman talk about her life-- her long 119-year-old life. It was comical to hear her discuss her medical problems and the arthritis that she had fought unsuccessfully for sixty-two years. She said she quit driving due to her arthritis as well as problems with her vision and hearing.

The professor then questioned how she had arrived at the hospital and she answered with a sweet smile, "Because I don't drive anymore, my young son brought me here. My little boy always helps to take me to all of my doctor appointments." Laughter could be heard throughout the room, because the little boy was a very friendly 97-year-old man. This little interview teaches us at least two points:

1. People can live considerably long lives.
2. Although there are many factors, it is possible that genetic factors could play a role in longevity.

Super-centenarians: What can we learn?

When experts direct studies of super-centenarians, a group of individuals characterized as being 110 years of age or older, the biggest question has been, "What we can learn from them?"

As of May 5, 2003, the membership of this very elite group numbered only forty-two. Thirty were women and twelve were men. Documenting the age of a super-centenarian is difficult; one can imagine the problem of maintaining accurate records of someone who has passed through different centuries. This group, who was born in the 19th century, lived through the entire 20th century and kept going into the 21st century. Incredible!!!

Experts are sure that we can learn much from them and apply the knowledge to our own lives. Perhaps the most important individual in that group of people is Madam Jeanne L. Calment from France who lived to be 122. Because the group is still very small and very diverse, it is too early to draw conclusions about what makes those people live so long. Thus far, we've not been able to attribute any specific factor as being responsible for the longevity in each one of these individuals. Recent studies show that a "genetic lottery," which is a unique situation when a very selective and specific group of genes fall into the right place at the right time, makes the difference in longevity rather than a lifestyle change. Although, we've definitely improved the quality and duration of our lives, there are no procedures, surgeries or medications available that could make an average person live that long.

> **Beauty by the Numbers**
>
> There are over 6 billion people in the world today, but only 60 are older than 110!

Even today, fifty years after Francis Crick and James Watson discovered the secret of life in the molecule of DNA; nothing can effectively be done to change our genetics to prolong life. Perhaps future genetic studies and advances in technology can change this picture.

Age, aging and rejuvenation

Before we continue to talk about aging, it is important to clarify a few definitions that are usually subjects of confusion. It is important to distinguish between *aging* and *senescence*. Aging is the time of life, counting in days, months or years and it is identical for everyone regardless of the life condition or the genetic background of the individual. Nothing can modify this process. Therefore, as hard as this may be for you to accept, if you are thirty-years-old, you will never be twenty again. Nothing can stop, slow, or reverse the clock. We all age in the same pattern.

Contrary to age, senescence is a rejuvenation process that can be modified and is very specific from one individual to another. Rejuvenation has to do with the process of aging and not the age itself. Rejuvenation has different meanings for doctors, patients or the companies that produce medications, cosmetics and other anti-aging products. These companies, motivated by dollar signs, typically make strong and sometimes misleading claims that the aging process can be reversed. Massive and aggressive marketing campaigns have forced us to believe this erroneous concept. However, one's appearance can be modified.

In a sense, youth can be manufactured. For example, if a forty-year-old woman underwent what we call medical rejuvenation procedures and treatments, she could possibly have the appearance of a thirty-year-old patient. This is the great mission of cosmetic medicine, particularly the ones that specialize in the aging process.

The Anti-aging Movement: Medicine of the 21st Century

Unfortunately, scientific studies show us that time is definitely not on our side. There is no question that time and aging cannot be stopped and to develop a true anti-aging medicine is impossible. However, the good news is there are things we can do.

I like to refer to anti-aging as "age management." How we manage our health is similar to how we manage our money. It doesn't matter how much money you have or what stage of your life you are in, you will need to manage your money well so you will not over live your assets. The same thing happens with your health. No matter how healthy or how old you are, you always do better if you can manage your health because you don't want to over live your health. You want to stay as healthy as possible, for as long as possible. Regardless of where you are or how you are, you need to manage.

It is essential to understand that aging is a natural process—not some horrid disease. Luckily, several dedicated medical specialists are available to make this process as smooth as possible for you.

Anti-aging, a new concept of medicine, works by combining all of the variables of your lifestyle such as health and the relationship with your environment to achieve and maintain a better and younger appearance. Anti-aging clinics attempt to collect and utilize current health data regarding preventive medicine and plastic surgery to allow their patients to look good as long as possible.

While you won't find an "anti-aging medicine" anytime soon, you should expect to find a growth in the number of clinics and doctors' devoted to help you in the process of age management. We now have at our fingertips new products, medications, and techniques to help improve the quality and duration of our lives.

What can you do?

My dad always used to say before you can help someone who is lost, you first need to find out where they are. Therefore, the first step of the anti-aging movement is to diagnose your aging and your speed of aging. Anti-aging is not about treating disease. Find a physician who specializes in anti-aging. General physicians are very good at treating diseases, but are horrible at maintaining health. To utilize anti-aging strategies, patients need to first find out where they're at. Not only do you need to know if you have any diseases, it's essential to find out where you are at in terms of nutrition. Also, how well are your hormones balanced? What screening tests have you taken? Just because you are disease free doesn't mean you are healthy.

A Piece of History

The original concept of "spa", which means to cure by water, is thought to date back to the Roman era. When warriors and land owners traveled, they'd need a place to rest if they became sick. Gladiators and warriors would stop to rest and restore themselves after battle. At these rest clinics, they could receive massages and good soup served with meat and vegetables. This, in fact, is also where today's name for "restaurant" came from. It was a popular belief that by feeding people, their health was being treated and maintained.

Much later, specific places were developed for restoring, massaging, feeding, and maintaining the health of people. Essentially, people were hosted here. Hence, we get the term "hospitalize" and "hospital".

As the Roman Empire fell, so did the popularity of the spa concept around the world. Existing spas were forgotten until they became transformed into vacationing hubs, losing their original purpose and catering only to the rich and famous. Other spas responded by focusing on the beauty business offering a variety of fitness and beauty services in glorified saloons called day spas.

Spas as we know today are emerging as centers for anti-aging, alternative medicines and have grown to include facials and massages.

The medicine of the future will focus on maintaining health, which I believe is much more cost effective if you consider that the United States spends over $1.3 trillion annually to treat disease. Health could be maintained among the same group of people for just a fraction of that cost. It's believed that for $300 billion, the health of the United States population can be maintained.

Clinics of the future will be places that will aid in managing your health. Although time is not on your side, there are many things that can be done. We can decrease the speed at which age occurs in our body and we can implement a contingent plan to deal with the things time has done to our body. Our body deterioration rate can be controlled to a certain degree just as you can control the aging of a piece of furniture or a car. The better the maintenance program you have, the better your goods can be preserved. This works for all your goods, including your body — the most precious asset of all.

✂ Dr. De Souza'a Beauty Secret ✂

Age is inevitable, but aging is not. Dr. DeSouza agrees that we won't live forever, but we should do everything we can to look good, feel good, and live as long as possible. The greatest part of this task is your responsibility. We need to take action for our own health. Doctors are very good at treating your diseases, but you are ultimately responsible for managing your health and not being sick to begin with.

Dieting, exercising, and living a healthy lifestyle are all part of your homework. Work hard and get an "A"!!

Chapter 4

Manufacturing Time

"God has given you one face and you make yourselves another."

-Shakespeare (1564-1616)

Facing your face

For Margaret Smith, it happened just like it does in the movies. It was one Saturday morning in 1963 and the children were with her ex-husband. It was one of those days that she used to call her "holiday". On Margaret's holidays, she took care of herself, ran some errands, and for a short period of time, she could be slightly selfish and think only about herself. When Margaret awakened, everything appeared to be normal— until she looked into the mirror. For some reason, a very strange feeling had overcome her. She found herself looking into the mirror and talking to herself. "I am fifty-years-old and I feel like I am forty, but I look like I am sixty," she told herself.

She wasn't quite sure how many thoughts raced through her mind in that second, but she saw a flashback of her entire life reflected in her face. Without any special reason, for the first time in her life, Margaret was facing her face in a completely different way than she normally did. On that particular Saturday morning, she viewed her face with a highly critical eye. She despised what she was looking at. She had bags under her eyes. She was horrified at how many wrinkles she had when she smiled and her whole face looked as if it were sagging. She felt that her face was loose with skin folds everywhere, particularly around the chin and jaw line.

Margaret Smith realized what millions of men and women around the world throughout history have also realized. As people grow older, the natural aging process aggravated by external factors such as sun exposure and weather takes a tremendous toll on one's facial appearance. The skin begins sagging and fitting more loosely with wrinkles, a double chin, and all the changes that are a common experience for everyone. Margaret suddenly longed for a more youthful appearance—in a sense, she wished she could manufacture time.

While there are no specific rules on how the aging process works, it is somewhat predictable. Because the face is the greeting card of the body--almost a picture of yourself and your personality--this change can be somewhat traumatic for people. It doesn't have to be so traumatic, however. Indeed, it is now possible to manufacture time as Margaret Smith wished for back in 1963. All that is needed is some skin repair and maintenance. After all, the body is a machine, and like any machine, maintenance needs to be performed regularly to keep it in tiptop shape.

It was exactly for this reason that in 1963, one procedure became the most important symbol of plastic surgery and facial rejuvenation, a procedure that we doctors call Rhytidectomy and is commonly known as the ***facelift***.

The first facelifts

It is not easy to ascertain when the first facelift was actually performed. In 1980, Dr. Rees attempted the difficult task of outlining the history of this fantastic and revolutionary surgical procedure.

However, the first documentation about facelifts definitely came from Europe and Germany. A surgery very similar to a facelift performed as it is performed today was described by Dr. Hollander in his book, *Handbuch Der Kosmetic*, which was published in 1912. It is very possible that Dr. Hollander performed the very first facelift on a polished aristocrat around 1901.

In 1906, Dr. Lexer also reported performing a revolutionary facial surgery on an actress. It is important to note that general anesthesia as we know it today was not available until the 1930's. With very little resources in anesthesia and surgical instruments, these doctors produced nothing but a miracle when performing cosmetic surgery under the primitive conditions at the beginning of the century. Apparently, the desire to be young and pretty overcame problems such as poor medical conditions and poor forms of anesthesia, pain control, and surgical instruments.

Anesthesia, surgery, and several other medical procedures related to cosmetic surgery experienced considerable development after World War II. At the beginning of the 1960's, facial surgery became an icon of facial rejuvenation; however, at this time it was reserved for movie stars and the rich and famous.

Over the past few decades, a wide range of new techniques and developments have been incorporated into the plastic surgery arsenal. Today, the process of manufacturing time is available to everyone and is no longer a single procedure.

The modern facelift

Currently, the facelift technique is a combination of different procedures that address different areas and different problems on the face. The aging process is a very complex process and surgeons today realize that the facelift should not be one procedure, but a combination of small procedures that can correct various problems in order to return a pretty and youthful face to the patient.

Nowadays, facelifts are considered to be a safe procedure that is also very popular. According to the Aesthetic Plastic Surgery Society, more than 117,000 cases of facelifts are performed every year in the United States alone.

It is a difficult mission for the physician to translate into medical terms what Margaret Smith saw when she looked into the mirror on that Saturday morning. Margaret knew that something was

The modern facelift is more than a simple surgery--it is a combination of art and science!

different with her face, however, that observation alone is not enough for a physician to be able to help the patient. In order to obtain good results with facial rejuvenation, it is necessary to have a detailed facial analysis.

More than a simple surgery

A very detailed process for facial analysis is described in *The Columbia Manual of Dermatologic Cosmetic Surgery,* written by Dr. Scarborough and Dr. Bisaccia. They analyze the intrinsic and extrinsic aging signs, and the process of aging through the years. They also recommend carefully evaluating the standards of beauty. What is beautiful to one person may not be beautiful to another person; therefore this analysis should be done with the patient. Finally, after the detailed analysis is completed, the doctor and patient agree on what needs to be corrected and what the goals are for the patient in that particular procedure. This added component makes the facelift a very unique procedure because it is not enough to simply discuss risks, benefits and post-surgical care as we would do with any other surgery. In this situation, we also need to discuss with the patient their desires, dreams and perceptions of beauty.

Once the facial analysis is conducted and the patient's complaints are clearly understood, a series of combined procedures should be planned. The overall program could involve tightening the facial and neck skin; tightening and pulling the facial and neck muscles;

removing excess skin and fat; elevating the eyebrows; and extracting wrinkles around the eyes, between the nose and mouth and on the forehead. Some patients require augmentation of the chin or even sealing of the wrinkles around the mouth and the eyes with collagen or fat. Liposuction can be used to remove fat in the areas of a double chin, and this fat can then be used to fill wrinkles and grooves throughout the face.

If desired, even plastic surgery of the nose and ears can be performed to help a patient return to grace, beauty and a youthful look. It is easy to understand how important the nose surgery is on the whole package of a facial rejuvenation. There is no question that the nose is the most prominent feature of the person's face. A small detail such as angle, size or curves on the nose can make a big difference in a patient's appearance. Large or big noses may give a person an old and angry face. A delicate nose with smooth and uplifted lines may give you a facial appearance of happy and young. Therefore, it is very common to combine nose surgery with a facelift to maximize results.

Less is more in the 21ˢᵗ century

If it were not enough to enjoy all the great successes and popularity of the facelift through the entire 20th century, the best was reserved for the end. In the last decade of the 20th century, new technology made this revolutionary procedure even more successful.

I remember the time when I was visiting the University of Alabama in Birmingham in 1990. I saw the great professor Vasconez and his disciples who had begun to explore some of the applications of the endoscopy techniques used in plastic surgery. At that time, it was just the initial clinical cases. However, there was no doubt that because of Dr. Vasconez and Dr. Saltz, endoscopy would play a very important role in the future of facial surgery and rejuvenation.

Endoscopic surgery has become a very popular procedure among surgical specialists, and it was no different with plastic surgery. Endoscopic procedures began to be used for treatment of facial fractures and small procedures. Now, it has become almost a standard of care for the rejuvenation of the upper part of the face.

The use of endoscopic surgery and facial rejuvenation has provided several advantages such as minimal scar formation, fewer traumas, less patient discomfort, and the possibility of performing the procedures under local anesthesia. This procedure is especially effective for elderly bald males as a large incision over the forehead is totally undesirable. A facelift can improve upper and mid-face features without a significantly large incision. This benefits the patient in a sense that it provides good results with minimal invasive surgery, and again in plastic surgery like any other in medicine, less is more. Fewer cuts represent fewer complications and faster recovery; Dr. Saltz and Dr. Core's studies show it clearly. In the new century, we feel the future is brighter for facial surgeries not only as a single procedure but also as a complex combination of several procedures trying to maintain or return balance, beauty and youth to the face.

Time for a facial tune-up

The biggest difference in this new century is in the surgery for facial rejuvenation. The timing of surgery will be of the utmost importance because it seems better for the patient to have a small combination of procedures at an early age rather than a big procedure at a later age. The biggest advantage to this new approach is the fact that one can do a small procedure under local anesthesia with less risk and with faster recovery that would not change one's appearance dramatically. Therefore, a person will be noticed as youthful and pretty, but nobody will notice the surgery. In the words of one of my teachers, Dr. Donnabella, the best facelift is the one that no one knows that you had.

For the future we envision a well-planned series of maintenance procedures for the skin to be performed starting in the second and third decades of life and continuing on throughout a patient's life. During the early stages of aging, in the second and third decade, the treatment is likely to be topical cream, skin restoration programs, and perhaps some laser, Botox injections, and very small in-office procedures.

As the patient progresses to the third and fourth decades, she will benefit from collagen injections, fat injections, repeated Botox injections, maintenance laser treatments to keep the skin healthy, hair removal, peeling, and using materials to fill in some of the deep wrinkles and grooves.

Finally, in the fifth or sixth decade of life, surgery will be necessary, but never as an old fashioned facelift with large incisions and large detachments of skin.

The treatment of the future will focus on specific areas, small incisions, and use of endoscopy to look inside the skin to pull the muscles into place. Muscles and ligaments will be repositioned in the face with minimal cuts, resections, less bruising, less pain and faster recovery. This program will be done in such a fashion that very few people will notice that the procedure was done, but many more people will notice that the patient looks prettier and younger. This process should be well understood by the doctor and the patient--it will be teamwork throughout life. The idea is more or less like taking your car in for a regular check-

Chapter 5

What is Beauty?

"Nothing makes a woman more beautiful than the belief that she is beautiful."

~ Sophia Loren   (1934 -)

Searching for beauty is nothing new. It seems to be a universal desire of the human race--this is unquestionable. What is questionable, however, is what exactly beauty is? How do you describe it? Despite the fact that an adequate and balanced physical structure is an important requirement for beauty to exist, a well-defined body structure does not define beauty.

What is considered today to be patterns of beauty are not always perfectly anatomical. In fact, it is not unusual to see people who are considered to be beautiful such as famous models and movie stars with less than perfect anatomy. Sometimes they are not symmetrical; sometimes their face presents irregularities in a way far from what we call a normal pattern, or perhaps some deformities are even present in such a unique way that they produce some interesting effects. Therefore, since beauty does not appear to be on the physical structure alone, what is it? What exactly is facial beauty? Defining beauty is a hard task. Scientists, philosophers, and doctors have tried to define beauty throughout the centuries, but most often without success.

If you happen to look in Webster's Dictionary, the definition for beauty is, "the quality in a person or thing that gives pleasure to the senses or pleasurable results to the mind or spirit." Well, that doesn't help very much, does it? There still remains the unanswered question--what is beauty? In an ideal world, we would have a universal definition of beauty that people of all ages and ethnic groups in various parts of the world could agree upon. They would agree upon which faces are attractive, and which are not. Research reveals several theories regarding why we consider some faces prettier than others.

In the 1800's, a British anthropologist and an American psychologist conducted a very interesting study. Sir Frances Galton and American George Stoddard composed portraits by superimposing photo exposures of several different faces. The results of the study both from Galton and Stoddard demonstrate that the canvases were better looking than the original picture itself, which suggests the theory that we as humans prefer an average face to a non-average face.

Self-perception

It is very intriguing that some people with a well-known pretty face do not see themselves as having a pretty face. They are always dissatisfied with their appearance. It is very common to see certain individuals as pretty, but that particular individual does not perceive themselves to be pretty. This phenomenon is very interesting and actually quite common. Patients from this group of people present a big problem for facial rejuvenation procedures. Several times they will look for a plastic surgeon or for cosmetic medicine to improve their appearance; and they are almost always unsatisfied with the results, even when the results are technically good. Why does this group of people not think that they are pretty? Why do they not perceive themselves as pretty, although everybody else does? What makes these people who are admired by everybody feel unattractive or sometimes even ugly?

"Beauty comes as much from the mind as from the eye."

~Grey Livingston

The Mona Lisa effect

There is another group of people who are even more interesting. Christine is one of the people in this fascinating group. There is no doubt that Christine is a very pretty woman; she always has been. She was elected prom queen, and she was always known for her beauty. Even now at forty-years-old and three children later, she is still a very attractive woman. Time has been relatively good to her. She also thinks she is pretty and she has no complaints except for one situation which she avoids as much as possible--being photographed. For some reason, Christine thinks that she has never looked good in a picture. She said in her own words, "There is no way. I do not do well in pictures; I'm not photogenic."

Christine belongs to this very interesting group of people known for their genes. The majority of the people consider people from this group beautiful. These people also consider themselves to be pretty, but they hate being photographed because they think that they never look good in pictures. They are never comfortable in front of a camera. They don't like to appear in photos, but at the same time they have no complaints about their appearance when they look in a mirror. The question is why does this group of people think that they do not look good on paper?

Three particular points compose our facial beauty.
   1) How do we see ourselves?
   2) How do other people see us?
   3) How we are actually?

These three perspectives should walk together in a very delicate and dynamic equilibrium. Otherwise, we will have a discrepancy between how you perceive yourself and how others perceive you. There are no scientific studies to explain why those people do not like their images in pictures. We simply call it the "Mona Lisa Effect."

Remember the structure of the face is comprised of more than thirty-six muscles functioning in very complex movements. Therefore, a patient can unconsciously modify the structure of their face and their appearance by moving different groups of muscles. When we change the position of the structure of the face, we change the points of light and shadows of the face.

According to Dr. Psillakis, when we involuntarily correct those possible imbalances of the face, we produce a more attractive face. This is a very subtle movement that the patient does without any consciousness of the act; however, it does produce a better appearance.

This subtle, yet complex modification of the facial structures can be very effective. Consider for example, when a photographer is photographing a model. The photographer knows that certain facial movements can change the appearance of the person being photographed. It is very common during professional photo sittings that the photographer requests the model to make specific faces related to specific emotions. The movements related to the requested emotion produce facial structure changes that would give the specific facial presentation. In some movements the face becomes more sexy or sad, and of course, beautiful. Beauty appears to be the combination of these important impressions.

It's essential that both the plastic surgeon and the patient be familiar with these aspects of beauty. Otherwise, the patient could be dissatisfied with their facial cosmetic treatment. In addition, being aware of this process also helps to develop appearances related to make-up and hairstyles.

What about you?

So how about you? To which group do you belong? Do you belong to Christine's group or do you belong to the group that doesn't think they are pretty although everyone else does? Maybe you are one of the lucky ones and you perceive your looks the same as everyone else does.

The best way to identify which group you belong to is to take a short trip through old family photo albums. If you happen to see several pictures of yourself that you do not like, then you probably belong to Christine's group. But all in all, it really doesn't matter which group you belong to.

Most importantly, you need to be aware and educated about these aspects of beauty. Increased knowledge of this process will allow you to improve yourself and to make necessary changes that you will find satisfying.

Dynamics of beauty

In addition to this great diversity of facial presentations, we should include the dynamics of beauty itself. Because the aging process is continuous, every day we are a different person—whether it be better or worse. It is only with the knowledge of your beauty that you will be able to maintain, improve or restore your beauty. Why is it so important to be pretty? Although studying or comparing beauty is not exactly a politically correct thing to do in America, we should not be naïve; we should recognize how important facial attractiveness really is. Along with intelligence and personality, facial attractiveness is critical to an individual's success.

Numerous behavioral, social, psychological, and anthropological studies have demonstrated the importance of attractiveness. The old adage, "Never judge a book by its cover," doesn't seem to apply to facial beauty. In several studies, children or adults demonstrate important rules of facial beauty as contributing to the overall success of the individual. There is no question that beautiful people have an advantage, and that advantage is present in every culture and at every age.

In her paper, *The Question of Beauty*, Dr. Judith Langlois describes a study performed on 150 Caucasian, Mexican, and African American newborn infants and their mothers. She describes that mothers of attractive firstborn infants were more attentive and affectionate than mothers of the less attractive firstborn. All mothers deny that attractiveness matters in parental treatment of the children, but their behavior ultimately contradicted their beliefs. Other studies described by Dr. Langlois demonstrate that facial beauty also has a significant correlation with children's popularity in the classroom.

Beauty is not in the eyes of the beholder

Within social relationships you are evaluated and there is no question that looking good has great benefits. However, the search for facial attractiveness is more than just looking good. Attractive people tend to have a higher quality of life provided that the other aspects of life are in equilibrium such as their health, personality, intelligence, relationships, etc. All things considered, it should be easy to understand that facial beauty is a very complex issue. Despite the numerous studies that have already been conducted, much more research will be necessary to help us define and understand beauty and the role it plays on human happiness and success. Thus far, evidence supports the idea that perception is not one, but actually a combination of at least three different aspects. Contrary to the famous saying, "Beauty is all in the eyes of the beholder," — the truth is that it probably isn't!!

Chapter 6

Facelift without Surgery

"You don't water the rose; you water the rosebush."

-Dr. Alex De Souza

E ven if you are healthy, you are going to age and eventually your skin will show it. However, there are things that can be done to repair, maintain, and protect your skin. When we talk about skin, we specifically mean the total body contour and structure. Beauty much more than just skin deep; it also involves muscles, bones, and etc.

It's important to understand the fact that some people are old, but don't think they are old. And then there are people who don't think they look old, but they are very old. Traditionally, if a person was not happy with their looks, they would have a surgical facelift, liposuction, a tummy tuck, etc.

Nowadays, however, people still want to look good, but they don't want the traditional facelift surgery that takes weeks to recover from. Instead, they are looking for noninvasive procedures with the least amount of pain and the least amount of down time as possible. Luckily, we live in a wonderful time where we have at our fingers, the highest quality of surgical procedures and anesthesia.

A Piece of History

In his book, *Handbuch Der Kosmetic*, Dr. Hollander reported performing a surgery very similar to the traditional facelifts that are performed today on a polished aristocrat in 1901.

Hmmm.....this is very interesting since general anesthesia as we know it today wasn't available until the 1930s!!

Is it possible to have a facelift without surgery?

A person's facial appearance is central to human interpersonal perception and is very often a testimonial of the aging process. Facial skin aging has classically been divided between biological aging (intrinsic aging) and extrinsic aging factors such as sun and environmental exposure. The clinical translation of that process is laxity, deepness of the expression lines, dryness and flatness of the dermal-epidermal interface with significant changes in the color, texture and overall quality of the skin.

Until very recently, it has been the belief that quality facial rejuvenation or body rejuvenation could not be obtained without major surgery. In 2004, a renowned group of surgeons from Philadelphia published a paper on facelift without surgery, asking the question: "Is it a fact or a myth?" The conclusion was that it was a myth—there was no way to obtain facelift results without surgery.

Now in 2009—only five years later—we can accurately say it *is* possible to achieve results that are comparable to a traditional facelift *without* subjecting the patient to a major procedure.

Through a combination of several new, noninvasive procedures that are customized for each patient, significant facial changes and a youthful and healthy appearance can be obtained without traditional surgical procedures.

Noninvasive lifts associated with skin restoration technologies such as laser, intense pulse light (IPL), radiofrequency, and new skin care delivery systems can indeed become the facelift of the future.

So how is it done?

The facelift without surgery is based upon two important points: The diagnosis of the aging face and a combination of two or more nonsurgical, minimally invasive techniques to obtain the desirable result.

Although a facelift without surgery is a fantastic approach because it is noninvasive, it is not quick. To achieve a facelift without surgery, approximately eight to twelve procedures are combined that span over a period of six to twelve months. Nevertheless, the patient has minimal disruption to their social and professional activities.

The process begins at the diagnosis level. First, the problem that the patient presents needs to be identified as well as the problems which seem to affect the patient the most. As a person ages, the bone structure absorbs and there is laxity of the soft tissue, the flesh, the general muscles, tendons, and skin. Therefore after time, a mismatch occurs between the bone structure and the soft tissue that covers the body. This mismatch not only occurs in the face, but also in the neck, hands, forearms, as well as throughout the entire body contour. This mismatch is generally responsible for the production of heavy wrinkles.

Although mismatch problems occur with varying intensity levels among different people, it is found that many people experience the following problems: discoloration of skin pigmentation, broken veins, redness, skin damage, and unwanted hair. In addition, it is common for the skin to become much thinner where there has been a disruption to the structure. This area has less collagen production and more elastin. Thinning skin causes the skin to lose its normal appearance and texture.

When the bone structure has become absorbed, there is generally a complete disruption of the natural contour of the face. Therefore, when a patient is approached, this factor must be taken into consideration. Not only is it necessary for the doctor to determine what the problem is, but he or she must also analyze what the patient's expectations are and give them what they want.

There are three vital steps to performing a facelift without surgery:

1) Skin repair and restoration, which every patient generally needs.

2) Skin tightening, which is often necessary; and

3) The thread lift, if necessary

Step One: Skin Restoration (The Christmas Gift Effect)

Believe it or not, a gift is only as good as its outward wrap. The first impression (even before you know what you are getting) you have of a gift is often by the way it's wrapped. A pretty Christmas wrap can make a huge impact on the person receiving the gift. The same concept can be applied to your looks. Consider your skin to be like Christmas wrap. If your skin has been damaged, take the time to repair it just as you would take the time to carefully wrap a Christmas gift. When you repair your skin, you repair your looks.

Skin restoration, which is typically performed in two stages, can be compared to remodeling kitchen cabinets. New cabinets cannot be hung until the old ones come down. Similarly, new skin cannot be brought out unless the old, dead skin on the top layer is first removed.

The restoration and repair process that we use is called "Skin Fitness." With Skin Fitness, skin damage is removed, skin is strengthened, and then the skin is maintained and protected.

When skin is repaired and a skin fitness program is implemented, serious health problems including skin cancer are actually being prevented.

Exfoliation

As stated earlier, the first step is to remove the damage and the old skin. If any type of cosmetic procedure is performed over dead skin, good results will not be achieved. Therefore, exfoliation becomes a key factor.

Microdermabrasion can be used to exfoliate but it's important that the correct microdermabrasion device is chosen in order to minimize trauma to the skin. If a patient has had a microdermabrasion treatment and is red and peeling a few days later, the treatment was too harsh. A good microdermabrasion should remove the dead skin without causing any redness or peeling.

After exfoliation is completed, and inflammation and oxidation is controlled, it is ideal to supplement the treatment with various compounds to control pigmentation and cell damage. One of the most important compounds for repairing skin is Retin A. Several studies have shown that Retina A can go inside the cells and correct DNA damage caused by the sun and prevent skin cancer. Because not all Retin A products are made equal, it's essential to select a product that has a delivery system that allows the products to be delivered inside of the skin. Otherwise the product is going to remain outside of the skin on top of the dead cells and there will be no response.

In addition to having pretty wrapping paper (good skin), you must also ensure that the wrap is tight. If the wrap is loose and doesn't cover the box nicely, then you will not have desirable results. In our house, it's a Christmas tradition to wrap gifts together as a family. You can usually tell which ones were wrapped by me and which ones were wrapped by my 8-year-old son. Although my son is very proud of his gifts, my gift wrapping tends to be a bit tighter than his. Just like our gift wrapping techniques, we must also tighten the skin around the bone structure of our face.

While there are numerous ways to accomplish the tightening of the skin, we actually try to shrink the skin by using a phenomena referred to as the "Blue Jean Effect."

Step Two: Skin Tightening – The Blue Jean Effect

As we age, there is a progressive mismatch between our bone structure and our flesh on our face and neck. I like to refer to this as the "Blue Jean Effect". Just as a pair of blue jeans stretch out and relax as we wear them; so does the flesh on our face and body. Have you ever noticed how much better jeans seem to fit after they've been washed and dried? This is because cotton, an organic fiber found in denim, shrinks after it has been heated in a dryer. Because our bodies contain a sophisticated organic fiber known as collagen, the same analogy can be applied to our bodies. Just as cotton shrinks when it is exposed to heat, collagen can also be made to shrink in the presence of heat.

Treatments such as range of frequency and lasers use heat to destroy, remodel, and shrink collagen around our face and body. This can produce a significant shrinking of the facial soft tissue and a better match with the facial bones. The patient is ultimately left with an improved facial contour, less droopiness, and less wrinkles. Although this sounds fantastic, simply tightening by heat is not enough.

WATER BALLOON PHENOMENA

Have you ever woke up in the morning to find that your eyes are puffy; but after you brush your teeth and eat breakfast, your eyes are fine? There happens to be a chronic collection of fluids in our bodies throughout our flesh that I refer to as the "water balloon phenomena." This phenomenon varies by degree from person to person. It also varies according to the time of day or stage of life we are in.

Water and sugar protein based products accumulate to produce swelling and a slush-like substance within our flesh. This is most evident when you wake up in the morning and see your puffy eyes and puffy face. After you've been awake for a while, your face returns to normal. The water essentially collects over night and then drains. This fascinating process varies among some females. Some women retain a lot of water during different phases of their menstrual cycle. Other women retain a lot of water due to certain medical conditions. One common condition that causes water retention is a low thyroid. People with low thyroid tend to have "mixeda," which is an accumulation of slush-like fluids within the fibers of our body.

Imagine a balloon that you fill with water. The balloon distends as its volume increases; it becomes heavier, and it drops. An empty balloon does not drop; in fact, it shrinks in volume. The same thing happens to our flesh. As the slushy substance is deposited within our flesh, our fibers distend so we gain volume in our face and throughout our body, which in turn disturbs our facial contour.

Until recently, there wasn't much that could be done to improve this condition. Some massage techniques have been developed for the purpose of draining the slush. The slush not only affects your looks, but it also affects your health by creating toxins that your body doesn't need. If allowed to accumulate long enough, the toxins can damage your cells. Therefore, to improve your looks and your health, your body should be detoxified to drain the slush.

THE TESLA TREATMENT

Because the plastic and cosmetic surgery fields are so dynamic, there are always new products and treatments being developed to help us with our problems. Tesla happens to be one of the most fantastic products we've ever been introduced to. Although simple, Tesla utilizes extremely high technology to deliver microcurrents throughout our body. Tesla uses microcurrent technology to perform lymphatic drainage and decrease the volume of fluid in our face and body. During this process of detoxification, signs of aging are decreased and the natural facial contour is improved. The Tesla treatment also improves oxygenation of the tissues. It is a well known fact that oxygen is the fuel of life and cells only function as good as the supply of oxygen is. Therefore, once your body is rid of the slush-like toxins, every cell in your body will function better. At the same time you improve your looks, you also improve the overall condition of your skin. When you control inflammation, you improve skin renewal and collagen formation.

By combining skin restoration and skin tightening techniques with accessory procedures such as the Tesla treatment, patients have the opportunity to obtain a much younger and healthier looking face. In the search for noninvasive procedures that are safe, painless, and has little downtime for the patient, the Tesla treatment offers big results with little effort.

IMPROVING YOUR "BOX"

As good as it sounds, nice wrapping paper on a gift is not enough. As you probably know from experience, it is much easier to wrap a gift that's in a box instead of one that is not in a box. The shape of the gift you are wrapping makes a big difference in the way the wrap looks. It doesn't matter if you use the prettiest or most expensive wrapping paper—if the shape of the gift is awkward, the wrap will not look good. Once again, this concept can be applied to your looks. Even if you have healthy, good-looking skin, it doesn't mean that your face will be pretty. It is essential that your facial shape—or box—be improved as well. So the better looking your "box" is, the better looking your Christmas gift will be.

Not only is the way a person's facial shape changes the No. 1 complaint about aging, it is also the No. 1 sign of aging. We know that when we improve the shape of the face, we are actually improving the "box." When the box is better, your wrap will be better, and consequently, your looks will be too. So for that purpose, we have the facelift.

Step Three: The Facelift

"Facelift" is a generic term that includes a large number of procedures that have the intent of restoring the shape of the face. Despite the connotation of the word "facelift," the procedure doesn't just involve lifting. A facelift involves lifting, wrapping, and improving the contour of the face. Basically, the term *lift* is used because most of the skin has to be repositioned due to the dropping of it as the skin ages.

The original roots of the facelift are difficult to track down, yet there are records of facelifts being performed more than 100 years ago. However, cosmetic facelifts only became a common procedure once we developed "good" medicine, which was toward the second half of the twentieth century.

A facelift is a very important part of the overall facial rejuvenation process, however, not all lifts are born equal. Over the last 20 years, I've witnessed the evolution of the facelift. During trips to Brazil, Barcelona, and Paris, I've been able to meet doctors who are making facelift history.

Starting in 1988, I had the pleasure of working with Dr. Psillakis and Dr. Vasconez for three years at the University of Alabama in Birmingham. Between 1988 and 1993, Dr. Psillakis created an amazing facial rejuvenation procedure called the subperiosteal facelift. Fantastic as this procedure was, though, it was quite invasive. Some patients even required hospitalization in the ICU. Needless to say, this type of procedure is becoming less and less acceptable.

A NEW DIRECTION FOR FACELIFTS

Using endoscopic procedures in other medical areas as a starting point, Dr. Saltz and Dr. Vasconez, also from Birmingham, Alabama, began working on facial rejuvenation procedures that were minimally invasive. Although endoscopic facelifts were much less invasive and less traumatic than the traditional facelift, it did not solve all the problems of the face. This is because facial muscles follow certain patterns that do not allow the endoscope to travel through it. Within the face, there is a significant amount of attachment between muscle, bone, and skin that traps the spaces. Endoscopic procedures tend to work better in the abdominal area because it is essentially just one big space, whereas in the face, there are several compartmental areas that will not accommodate an endoscope.

For the parts of the face where an endoscope cannot be effectively used, several other lift techniques have been developed such as the Smart lift and Minilift. These type of procedures attempt to decrease the number of incisions made on the flesh, however, cuts around and behind the ear are still necessary and are usually noticeable. These visible incisions sometimes contribute to the stigma of the facelift. Ideally, we would like procedures that don't require incisions and don't leave scars. For this reason is why the thread lift has become a favorite.

The Thread Lift

The thread lift, a very popular procedure among cosmetic surgeons, is not new. In fact, the idea of using thread to lift and support facial skin has been around since the 1970s.

The problem with the original thread lifts is that the procedure, which used surgical or gold thread to pull the skin back and up over the skull, did not always hold and eventually, the sutures would rip or dissolve. Sutures would also float to the surface of the skin causing an asymmetrical appearance. Bunching effects would also sometimes appear above the hairline requiring that the entire string be removed.

Unlike a traditional facelift where the patient is usually under anesthesia, the patient is awake during a thread lift. This allows the client to hold a mirror to see if he or she is satisfied with the results. If not, the thread can be pulled tighter or let looser to achieve the desired look.

The procedure is fairly comfortable and only requires a two to three day recovery time. Another benefit is that unlike a conventional facelift, the patient has the gratification of seeing the results immediately.

I'm quite certain that facelifts of the future will be centered on thread-based techniques. It is difficult if not impossible to rejuvenate a face without lifting up structures that may have fallen; therefore, some sort of facelift will be essential.

Beauty by the Numbers

Since 1997, there has been a 457 percent increase in the total number of cosmetic procedures. Surgical procedures increased by 114 percent, and nonsurgical procedures increased by 754 percent.

*According to the American Society for Aesthetic Plastic Surgery

---

The Invisible Lift

Because of the problems encountered with older thread lifts, doctors try to use material which will hold for a long time and which will also be well tolerated by the patient's body. In addition, doctors prefer to use a thread technique that looks as natural as possible.

Since its inception six years ago and over 300 cases performed, the *"Invisible Lift"*, a simple outpatient procedure, offers the best of both worlds. By using the Invisible Lift, we try to combine the benefits of the conventional facelift with a thread lift. The idea is to perform a procedure where results last for a reasonably long time, results can be reproduced and the procedure is safe and comfortable for the patient. During an Invisible Lift, no cuts or incisions are made and only local anesthesia is used.

Through a small needle hole, we are able to pass a thread around the muscles of the face and then pull it tight to give the appearance of a facelift. Unlike a traditional facelift, a patient can see results immediately.

Scientific studies indicate that the results of a thread lift are quite similar to those of a traditional lift. Because the Invisible Lift has only been performed for approximately six years, it's too early to determine just how long the results will last. Just as a conventional facelift loses results with time, it is fair to ascertain that the Invisible Lift and other modern thread lifts won't last forever either. But patients are always better off reaping the benefits of a facelift than not having one at all.

Facelift: Success or Failure?

What may be a successful surgery in the eyes of a doctor may not always be successful to the patient. From a surgeon's point of view, a successful surgery is one where the patient wakes up from the anesthesia and the incisions heal well without any infections. Strange as it may sound, these are not top priorities for the patient. The most important thing to the patient is how they think they look. It doesn't matter if the surgeon and everybody else think the patient looks great. It's what the patient thinks; it's what they see when they look in the mirror. Perception is everything to them.

With a traditional facelift, if a patient looks in the mirror and hates the way they look, there is nothing that can be done. The surgical results are permanent. However, results are 100% reversible with the Invisible Lift. If the patient doesn't like what they see, the procedure can be undone.

As I've progressed in my career, I've learned many, many things. But perhaps one of the most valuable lessons I've learned is that the overall facial rejuvenation process is extremely complex because the emotional charge attached to it is tremendous.

In my opinion, patients not only want to look younger, they want their *own* youth back. Therefore, it's critical that doctors avoid altering the look of their patients so much that they are unsatisfied with the results of the procedure. There are serious psychological consequences associated with facelifts when a patient's appearance is changed so much that they do not look like themselves.

Regardless if a person is fat, ugly, young, or old, we are the person that we love the most. If we make significant changes to a patient's appearance or do not give them back *their* youth, the patient will be unsatisfied with the surgery.

The challenges of plastic surgery are quite unique. After gall bladder surgery, you expect that you will no longer be sick, that your gall bladder will be gone and that you will have a scar on your abdominal area. But with a facelift, it's important to remember that the patient wasn't even sick to begin with. They went to the doctor for a procedure that they didn't even need. Then they suddenly come away looking completely different. It is a very frightening idea for most people.

Our program, Optimal Health, is designed to be gradual, gentle, and manageable to allow patients the time to make decisions. More freedom is given to the patients to obtain the results they want. Through our Optimal Health program, we repair, tighten, and lift the skin as well as address the patient's overall health so they feel and look better.

Other Accessory Treatments

In addition to the three major steps discussed, a facelift without surgery also includes accessory treatments which help to maximize the results of facial rejuvenation. Common procedures such as liposuction help to obtain a better contour. Liposuction, which started out to be extremely invasive, can now be performed in a minimally invasive manner on an outpatient basis using only local anesthesia. Liposuction is helpful for removing unwanted fat and improving the body's contour.

Collagen fillers help to create smooth facial skin while decreasing wrinkles. The most commonly used cosmetic procedure throughout the world is the botulinic toxin, which is very effective in helping limit movement in the eye and forehead area. Muscle control is extremely important in the overall package and has a tremendous effect on the appearance of the face as well as the prevention of wrinkles.

Although some people prefer not to use the botulinic toxin because they consider it to be a toxin, we suggest administering it in small doses two or three times a year because it can help with muscle control. It's important to realize that we have 37 muscles in our face that are constantly moving as we smile, talk, chew and blink (believe it or not, we blink about 18,000 times a day). Because the skin lies directly over the facial muscles, the constant movements or muscle action causes significant skin damage and wrinkles. Therefore, during the facial restoration process, we need to control the muscle action by decreasing the muscle action to improve the wrinkles.

RESHAPING WITH BIOPLASTY

Just as Botox® revolutionized the way that we treat facial wrinkles, I'm convinced that bioplasty will revolutionize the way we treat facial contouring and facial rejuvenation. Bioplasty is a term created about 20 years ago by Dr. Nacul, a plastic surgeon from Brazil. Dr. Nacul describes the bioplasty procedure as one that allows physicians to reshape the facial structures to restore its youth and beauty.

Dr. Nacul refers to bioplasty as "interactive" plastic surgery because the patient is completely awake during the procedure (while holding a mirror) and therefore has full control of the "sculpting" process.

While several different fillers have been utilized in bioplasty procedures, the most commonly used filler is called *polimetilmetacrilate* or PMMA.

Dr. Nacul uses PMMA for reshaping the face and for body contouring. In some cases, PMMA has been used with excellent results to treat patients with facial deformities or trauma injuries.

Although bioplasty has only been approved for use in the United States since 2006, I believe it will become one of the most popularly performed procedures. Bioplasty, a safe and minimally invasive procedure, has been successfully performed on over a million patients in more than a dozen countries. In Brazil, where there are more than 80,000 new bioplasty patients each year, more than 2,000 plastic surgeons perform the procedure on a daily basis.

Now that the FDA has approved the bioplasty procedure in the United States, we can expect the number of bioplasty patients to increase even more. Bioplasty allows doctors to reconstruct facial and body contours much more effectively. In the past, fillers were primarily used for correcting deep facial wrinkles, but now we can use PMMA to actually rebuild areas of the face. Although reconstruction has been tried with other fillers in the past, PMMA offers patients a more natural appearance with a more natural feel.

Bioplasty is just one more way that allows us to do more for less!

PMMA Facts

- Polimetilmetacrilate (PMMA) was discovered in Germany in 1902, by the chemist O. Röhm and was patented in 1928.
- PMMA was first used for health purposes in 1936. It has been intensively utilized since then in a variety of medical and odontological products.
- PMMA has been used as bone cement, knee implants, intraocular implants.
- In 1989, G. Lemperle first used PMMA as an injecting product for tissue. Since then, PMMA has been used as injecting implant in more than two million patients with stability, excellent results and minimal complications.
- PMMA is a biomaterial approved by the US Food and Drug Administration (FDA).

Final Advice

One thing that I've learned during my 25 years of work is that the patient does not want to simply look young again; they want their *own* youth back. Very often you will see a movie star who has gotten a traditional facelift. While they do look younger, they do not look like themselves. They look pulled and stretched.

Having a cosmetic procedure is a very personal issue. One of the main advantages of a facelift without surgery is that it is much easier to obtain the patient's desired results.

For the first time, by combining a host of new techniques and procedures, a truly nonsurgical facelift exists. This quite affordable procedure offers good results, without any stitches and cuts or downtime, allowing the patient to resume normal activities immediately. And unlike traditional surgical facelifts, the new Invisible Lift is 100% reversible.

If a patient is unhappy, we can remove the threads yet they still have the benefits of the skin tightening and skin repair. Skin tightening and repair procedures are excellent because they improve the health of the skin and improve your appearance without major changes. The lift merely complements those procedures.

If the clock cannot be slowed, at least you can have the opportunity to obtain an appearance years young than you really are. Through an innovative approach of combining customized facial restoration procedures, it is possible to "manufacture time."

🌿 Dr. De Souza's Secret 🌿

People certainly want to look better, but with life as it is today, it is very difficult—even for the rich and famous—to undergo a major procedure such as a conventional facelift.

Luckily, we now live in an era where facial skin rejuvenation can be done without surgery and is based on three steps:

Step 1- Skin restoration

Step 2- Skin tightening

Step 3- Facial reshaping, where we use lifts and combinations of lifts.

The more skin repair procedures you combine, the better results you will have. The less invasive the procedures are the more comfortable and natural the results will be. So, the next time you are considering facial rejuvenation, think about noninvasive procedures as well as a combination of them. It is impossible to improve one physical feature 100 percent, but you can improve a lot of features by 80 percent and get much better results.

Skin cannot be repaired from outside in only. It must also be repaired from the inside out. Therefore, the building blocks for good skin include being well- nourished, well-hydrated, and having well-balanced hormones.

Chapter 7

The Good, the Bad, and the Ugly

"Anyone who says sunshine brings happiness has never danced in the rain."

~Author Unknown

Sun tanning is by far the good guy of the story. There is something special about being tanned, but what is it? When did this entire tanning obsession start? Until the end of the 19th century, sun exposure was linked to the poor and the lower social class. Since nobility and the rich did not need to work outdoors, they were never exposed to the sun and consequently never had a suntan. Their skin was so fair that one could see their bluish veins underneath; it was common to hear the families of the rich as well as the nobility called "blue blood individuals." However, everything changed with the turn of the century.

> **Did You Know?**
>
> Used in some rural areas of the United States, the term "red neck" was originally given to an individual with significant sun exposure. It took many, many decades for a person with a suntan to be seen as fashionable.

It wasn't until the 20th century that tanning became associated with beauty, success, and leisure. The first two decades of the 20th century marked the use of sun exposure for wellness treatments such as anemia, fatigue and even tuberculosis. Without antibiotics or any other effective means of treatment, very little could be done for chronic infections. At the beginning of the century, sun therapy or sunbaths were a mandatory part of the tuberculosis program all over the world.

From disease to health and then on to the French Riviera, sun tanning reached fashion shows all over the world. It's believed that the French fashion designer, Gabrielle Coco Channel, recognized the suntan as a sign of beauty and health. With the development of colorized movies, the idea spread even more among the models and movie stars; and they desired to be tan.

Despite well-known risks, the suntan is still very popular. Every single day, approximately one million Americans use tanning beds and millions enjoy the natural sunlight. The suntan is no longer a sign of nobility but a sign of health, energy and fitness. Exercise, sports and action are also associated with a suntan. Who doesn't remember Elvis Presley's movies on the beach or the hot tunes from the Beach Boys such as "Surfing Safari, Surfin' USA" that hit the top of the charts in the 1960's?

In the 1970's, the association between beauty and suntans became even clearer. Actress Farrah Fawcett's tanned face and sparkling white smile became a popular symbol of sensuality and beauty. A few years later, Bo Derek brought the glamour of suntan to the entire body. Finally, against medical advice, men and women still insisted on searching for a tan simply because they liked it. One day, the famous model, Christy Turlington, was questioned why she tanned and she said, "Just because..." If people still want a suntan, the question is how to tan the skin with as little risk as possible.

Sunlight- good or bad?

A Piece of History

French clothing designer Coco Chanel can be credited blamed) for the transformation from pale skin to tan skin. In 1920s, as Chanel was designing more liberal women's fashions, inadvertently gave the fashion world another new trend. Wh cruising from Paris to Cannes aboard the Duke of Westminst yacht, she obtained a suntan--probably by accident!

Is sunlight good for you? Yes, it is—but only to an extent! It feels good, improves people's moods and energy levels, plus it aids in the production of Vitamin D, which helps to build strong bones. Therefore, moderate sun exposure does have other benefits besides a great looking tan. Nevertheless, these benefits do not come without a lofty price. Excess sun exposure accelerates the aging process and can cause such serious skin damage such as wrinkles, dark spots, and skin cancer.

The sunlight has several different radiation levels with infrared and ultraviolet (UV) being the most important ones, particularly the UV. UV can further be divided into UVA, UVB and more recently UVC, which has been a cause of concern. One of the functions of the ozone layer is to protect us against sun radiation, but as the ozone layer becomes damaged, UVC rays are able to pass through therefore causing significant damage to the skin. All UV rays have the potential to damage the cells of our skin and unfortunately, that damage is permanent. Our body can do very little to protect us from that damage.

Skin Color and Skin Types

The skin is a very complex organ and every individual has a different type of skin. Due to the large variety of genetic presentation and the relationship, it is difficult to clearly classify different types of skin; however, the studies from Dr. Fitzpatrick in the 70's and 80's offer us a classification that was originally intended for determining tanning ability and photo aging.

Today, Dr. Fitzpatrick's classification of the skin comes in a universal language for plastic surgeons, dermatologists, cosmetic medicine and all doctors involved with skin care. Despite the fact that there are other classifications, we all use Dr. Fitzpatrick's scale of tanning ability as a classification of the skin. This classification includes six types of skin ranging from Type I to Type VI. While many other classifications have been used, the Fitzpatrick scale has been used as the universal language for skin types.

Dr. Fitzpatrick's scale of tanning ability

- **Type I**-- patient is of white skin, light hair and light eyes, the one that never tans quickly and becomes red under sun exposure.
- **Type II**--rarely tans and remains with a very low threshold of sunburn.
- **Type III**--is in between, sometimes burns mildly but usually tans.
- **Type IV**--is usually a dark skin – classically the Hispanic or Asian patient with dark hair and dark eyes but still sunburns if exposed long enough.
- **Type V**-- is a progression of that scale.
- **Type VI**-- is the opposite of Type I – the patient usually has dark hair, dark eyes, and even darker skin with no problems with redness.

Photo aging classification

A universal classification system for photo aging was developed by Dr. Glogau and is another system that doctors use for predicting outcomes of sun exposure. Glogau ranks the capacity of damage to the skin from the sun according to groups that range from one to four. By using both Fitzpatrick and Glogau's classifications, a doctor would be able to tell you your risks of exposure to sunlight, to tanning beds, and also the risks for development of skin cancer. We can also determine if a patient is a suitable candidate for different types of cosmetic procedures, if complications such as a tendency for unpleasant cosmetic scars will arise, and even how the aging process can affect you depending upon your type of skin.

Dr. Glogau's Photoaging Classification System				
Group	Classification	Typical Age	Description	Skin Characteristics
I	Mild	28-35	No Wrinkles	Early Photoaging: mild pigment changes, no keratosis, minimal wrinkles
II	Moderate	35-50	Wrinkles in motion	Early to Moderate Photoaging: Early brown spots visible, keratosis palpable but not visible, parallel smile lines begin to appear
III	Advanced	50-65	Wrinkles at rest	Advanced Photoaging: Obvious discolorations, visible capillaries (telangiectasias), visible keratosis
IV	Severe	60-75	Only wrinkles	Severe Photoaging: Yellow-gray skin color, prior skin malignancies, wrinkles throughout - no normal skin, cannot wear makeup because it cakes and cracks

How does our skin change color?

The color of the skin itself comes from a pigment called melanin. The melanin is produced by one specific type of skin cell called melanocytes. When UV rays are stimulated, melanocytes are activated and produce more melanin, which is the skin pigment that gives color to our eyes and to our skin. Melanin gives your skin its natural color as well as the tan. UV rays from the sun changes the already existent melanin and stimulates the production of further melanin. That is why you tend to look darker after you leave the beach or tanning bed. Because your body continues to produce and make changes in the melanin, your tan can still get darker for hours after you leave the exposure site of the UV light.

The tan you receive is visible proof that the skin is being heated by the UV light. Therefore, despite the pleasant appearance of the sun tan, it is nothing other than skin damage in disguise. No matter what type of skin you have, suntans still damage your skin and you still run the risk of getting skin cancer.

Biological aging vs. the aging process

Skin cancer isn't the only thing to worry about when it comes to the effects of UV light on the skin. Studies indicate that aging signs can be accelerated or modified by more or less exposure to the sun. It is important to differentiate, however, between *biological aging,* which is a natural process of the skin that becomes thin and weak, and the *aging process*, which is the result of sunlight exposure.

With the aging process caused by sun exposure, the skin tends to become thicker and almost yellowish-gray in color. Also, the skin is frequently red with visible scabby areas and significant changes occur in color and texture, which gives the skin a leathery appearance — a very typical look for individuals who have a long history of sun exposure. In addition to all these changes, the skin can have an undesirable appearance caused by multiple areas of broken veins that are visible underneath the skin, brown aging spots, freckles on the skin, uneven skin tone, saggy skin looking older than it is, and plenty of wrinkles!!

All suntans are not created equal

Although sun tanning seems to be most popular among young females, people of all ages seem to enjoy it. For some time now, there has been a great deal of conflict between the cosmetic industry and the medical community. On the one hand, the cosmetic industry uses strong marketing strategies to sell their suntan-related products, and then on the other hand, the medical community is concerned due to well-known damage of the human body caused by ultraviolet radiation (also known as UV rays).

Millions of dollars are spent on research every year to find a safe tan. So far, there is no such thing as a safe tan. All tanning techniques are the same, and the most common is the suntan from the natural sunlight.

Tanning Bed Precautions

Should you still desire to use a tanning bed, be sure to take the following precautions:

- Be sure to visit your doctor prior to using the tanning bed to discuss with him which type of skin you have. The type of skin you have is very important because a burn is very damaging to the skin and a tan is what you are looking for. Some types of skin only burn and do not tan.
- Limit your exposure time to the minimum adequate for your skin type. If you cannot avoid the tanning bed, you should have small exposures for a long period of time; that way your skin is more prepared to respond.
- Have skin moles and other lesions on the skin examined before any kind of sun exposure or a tanning bed session.
- With your pharmacist and/or doctor, review any medications that you may be taking in order to avoid a possible skin reaction. Certain medications can increase the sensitivity of the skin to the sun, so many physicians advise patients to avoid sunlight or tanning bed exposure while taking them.
- Use sun block and use eye protection – protecting the eye is very important. In twenty-nine states, the Federal Trade Commission requires tanning salons to request that customers use protective eye wear. Moderation is the magical word when it comes to tanning beds. Fifteen to twenty minutes in a tanning bed is just about equivalent to spending a full day at the beach.

Tanning Bed

To satisfy the demands for tanned skin, a popular device known as the tanning bed was created. Initially, it was a great success in Europe and by 1975; it started to gain popularity in America. Today tanning beds are so popular that some cities have more of them than they do ATM machines. Despite the fact that tanning bed radiation can provide some physical and psychological health benefits, the majority of the medical literature agrees that tanning beds not represent a safe tanning option. Although UV radiation differs from bed to bed, they usually contain less UVB and significantly more UVA than the natural sunlight. This leads to less sunburn, but not safe tanning because with time, the UVA rays alters skin in such a way that it too, could lead to skin cancer.

UV radiation produces free radicals, which can directly damage the DNA (the most important part of our cells). In a short period of time, UV causes damage and produces a painful burn. Over a long time, it causes premature aging, and unfortunately, millions of cases of skin cancer are diagnosed in America every year.

It's true that visits to a tanning bed can be beneficial for diseases such as vitiligo and psoriasis, and it can increase energy levels, and helps to strengthen bones with the production of Vitamin D. While the amount of radiation exposure can be controlled within a tanning bed environment and can't be done with the sun, these benefits do not outweigh the associated risks.

Several dermatologists agree that safeguards are not enough to protect your skin from damage. One needs to remember that the tanning bed is a $5 billion industry with tremendous marketing material trying to convince us that there is less risk with tanning beds than with sunlight itself. This is a story much like the one regarding tobacco – there is no such thing as safe smoking. If you decide to go for a tan, be sure that you are well educated about the risks and try to minimize exposure as much as possible.

Tan in a pill

In an attempt to resolve the dilemma between having a tanned look and avoiding suntan risks, the cosmetic industry and the medical community have been working hard to develop methods for sunless tanning. Since the 1960's, several drugs have been developed in an attempt to create a sunless tan. In particular, one drug is dihydroxyacetone or simply DHA. This drug contains the only active ingredient approved by the FDA for sunless tanning. DHA interacts with the proteins on the outer layer of skin and produces a darkening effect.

This is an important product giving one the cosmetic effect of a suntan without the damage of the sunlight or the radiation of a tanning bed. It can also help patients with medical problems such as vitiligo, albinism and other diseases that tend to change the color of the skin. Although it is not perfect, at least it can give you some degree of a tanned look.

Despite persuasive advertisements, the tanning pills that you've probably heard about contain products such as carotenoids, fruits, vegetables and flour products. The most common one has chemicals derived from pre-Vitamin A that could produce a yellowish-brown skin; however, these products are not approved by the FDA and should not be used due to dangerous side effects that could possibly occur.

Tan in a bottle

Other products on the market promise to give what people call a "Tan in a Bottle." Most of these products have DHA plus other medications. They also help give the skin a more natural, suntanned appearance, but a perfect sunless tan is still not available. In the next few years we can probably expect to see great improvement in the area of sunless tanning products.

Unfortunately, not even the tan in a bottle is a safe alternative to the sun due to the fact that it is made of several chemical elements. Depending upon your skin type, a skin reaction, allergic reaction or other problems can occur. As mentioned before, it's important to seek medical advice before using any type of tanning method.

Although we finished the 20th century and the ideal sunless tan is yet to be created, the medical community places its hope in this type of tan because it is the only one that does not carry the skin cancer risk.

> **Beauty by the Numbers**
>
> It is important to understand that the SPF of a sunscreen indicates the length of time that the product gives protection from the sun and not necessarily the strength of the product. SPF 15 is not three times as strong as SPF 5—it just lasts three times longer!!

The Birth of Sunscreen

During the most difficult days of World War II and the hottest summer days in the South Pacific, the last thing that was probably on the mind of our embattled soldiers was getting a sun burn. Nevertheless, imagine our fair-skinned men skin spending many hours fighting in the hot sun on the sun-drenched beaches of the South Pacific while their skin was getting scorched. Although a war was being fought, it was in this harsh environment that the first modern sunscreen was born.

Benjamin Green, an airman, was part of the team that developed a special formula that was applied to the skin of soldiers to protect them on the battlefields and on the ships. It was a strange-looking cream that had a strange-sounding name, "Red vet pet." The soldiers used the petroleum-based ointment to protect their skins from the sun. Because of the sticky nature of the product, it earned the nickname of "red goo".

Green later became a pharmacist and in 1944, he used his invention to develop the first commercial product for sunburn protection. Green's product was later known as Coppertone Suntan cream. It was the first sun care product to be sold to regular customers. When Green and his wife improved the original mix by adding cocoa butter and jasmine, the old red goo became much more tolerable. Nevertheless, it is fair to consider the red goo that our soldiers used as the father of all sunscreens. When the men returned home from war, several of them had acquired the habit of using sun protection; thus making sunscreen very popular.

In the 50's and 60's, we learned a great deal about sun protection. The discussion about risks and benefits of sun tanning versus sun protection continued until 1979, when the FDA concluded that sunscreen would be helpful in preventing skin cancer. During last two decades of the 20th century the extensive knowledge about skin, skin function, and the nature of the sun's radiation, defined the need to protect our skin much more effectively.

In 1980, Coppertone developed the first sunscreen product that included protection from the UVA and UVV at the same time. Wearing a long-sleeved shirt, long pants or skirts and even a hat can reduce skin damage today from radiation. In addition, the use of a comprehensive program of skin care to maintain the health of the skin by proper protection using sunscreen will help to prevent photo-damage. Nevertheless, the only truthful way to avoid problems is to avoid the sun. The tan itself is visible proof that the skin is being damaged. Therefore, it is impossible to have a tan without damage to the skin.

Sunscreens 101

There are different types of sunscreen. The effectiveness of the sunscreen product is indicated by a ratio known as sun protection factor or SPF. SPF is the amount of additional time a person can stay in the sun before they may burn, as opposed to a person with no sunscreen protection. For example, an SPF of 20 indicates that a person could remain outside twenty times longer than a person without sunscreen and sustain the same burn level. Sunscreens are available with SPF levels up to 50, but an SPF of 15 to 30 is typically sufficient, as an SPF of 10 will block 90% of UVB rays.

Obagi Skin Classification System

Skin Variable	Pre- and Postprocedure Skin Conditioning	Suitable Procedures and Potential Reactions to Procedure	Postprocedure Management
Color	Darker skin: Aggressive conditioning before procedure and after healing to minimize PIH	Hypopigmentation • Light procedures:rare • Medium-depth procedures:possible Hyperpigmentation:common • More likely	Dark skin: Condition aggressively to minimize PIH
Oiliness	Interferes with effectiveness of preprocedure conditioning.	Topical treatment needed to reduce surface oil prior to procedure.	Interferes with effectiveness of postprocedure conditioning. Topical treatment needed to reduce surface oil.
Thickness	Thick skin needs correction and stimulation; thin skin needs more stimulation.	Thick skin: best for chemical peels, dermabrasion Medium-thick skin: best for TCA peels, dermabrasion, CO_2 laser Thin skin: lighter procedures such as Blue Peel; erbium resurfacing	Correction and stimulation as needed
Laxity	Long-term stimulation to prevent further laxity	Skin laxity: medium-depth peel or several Blue Peels are ideal Muscle laxity: face-lift, alone or combined with a Blue Peel to correct associated skin laxity, may be needed.	Correction and stimulation, as needed.
Fragility	Aggressive stimulation to strengthen the skin	Correlates with postsurgical scarring. In fragile skin, procedure depth should be limited to papillary dermis	More cycles of correction and stimulation, as tolerated

Besides the factor, some sunscreens protect against UVB and others against UVA or both. Some chemical agents physically block the UV light as in the case of zinc oxide or titanium dioxide. Those products are called sun blocks due to the efficient block of the UV light. These two sun blocks as described earlier can scatter, reflect or absorb all the UV light; therefore, they are better protection and are waterproof. Zinc oxide has been described as the chemical choice to produce such a type of sun block.

Final Advice

If the suntan is good and the sunburn is bad, there is no question that skin cancer is the ugly one. It reminds me of a patient of mine who is six years old that brought me a drawing about cancer and his definition of cancer was ugly. Until a couple years ago, I had that drawing in my office; I always remember him when I talk about cancer. Ugly is a very good word to describe what it is.

The number of skin cancer cases has increased to over one million every year, and skin cancer claims more than 10,000 lives every year in the United States alone. While there are several factors that contribute to skin cancer, there is no question that sun exposure is the number one avoidable cause of the disease.

It's crucial to note that skin damage is for life. When we observe skin damage or skin cancer in a 70-year-old patient, many times it was due to a process that happened when the patient was a child, years and years before. That shows how important it is for parents, educators, and day care centers to take the responsibility to protect children from the sun in order to avoid a problem for life.

☙ Dr. De Souza's Secret ❧

If you can't avoid the direct exposure of the sun or the tanning bed, please be sure that you use all the protection you can afford. By avoiding tanning, you avoid future problems and your skin will thank you for it. Knowing your skin type will help you decide how long you can expose yourself to the sun without burning or how long to be in the tanning bed without damaging your skin. The good, the bad, and the ugly show the difficult balance between looking good, looking fashionable and being healthy.

Chapter 8

Body Rejuvenation

"Take care of your body. It's the only place you have to live!"

~Jim Rohn

Traditionally, facial rejuvenation has been at the front line of the battle against aging in our body. There is no question that the rest of our body suffers from the same aging process as our faces. Needless to say, the demands for body rejuvenation procedures are very high.

At the same time the facelift was developed, procedures for enhancing other parts of the body were also developed. These procedures include the tummy tuck, liposuction, and treatments for the leg and arm. Even procedures for hands and feet have become increasingly popular.

In the same way that people want noninvasive procedures for the face, they also look to those types for the rest of the body. We can perform surgeries today that we could never perform before. If you were to ask 10 people, most likely, they would all prefer procedures that do not require general anesthesia or any downtime. Many times people can't afford to take four to six weeks off to recover from a facelift.

In the future, you will see a dramatic shift from major surgical procedures to multiple noninvasive surgeries. I believe that we will not perform major surgical procedures in the future and the trend that we now see in noninvasive facial rejuvenation procedures will also carry over to the rest of the body.

However, some of the body rejuvenation surgeries that have been traditionally in high demand will continue to be used for some situations. But more and more, patients are starting to take care of the aging process early on. Fortunately, when the diagnosis of the aging process is made early, the chances for success using noninvasive procedures are much higher.

> **Did you know?**
>
> The number of muscles in the human body varies from about 656 to 850, depending on which expert you consult. No exact figure is available because there are a variety of opinions about what constitutes a distinct muscle (versus a part of a complex muscle). Also, there is some variability in muscular structure between individuals.

Aging Process of the Body

The anatomical and physiologic change that happens to our face also happens to our body. The bone structure that supports our body undergoes a dramatic change caused by aging. There is the absorption of the bone and the shrinkage of the backbones, which affects our posture, our height, and the way that our body is supported. At the same time that the bone structure becomes weak and shrinks, the muscles throughout our body become placid and lose their toneness, which results in a drop of the structures. This change is particularly noticeable on the back of the arms and on the thighs.

Throughout the entire body, we see a decrease of muscle toneness and positioning. Just as the soft tissues of the face are affected with laxity and there is a drop of skin envelope, a mismatch also occurs between our soft tissues, skin, and muscles, which ultimately cause the complaint of sagging skin on our arms, legs, and abdominal area.

"The body never lies."

~Martha Graham

At the same time the muscle loses its tone, and the bones decrease in volume and size, fat deposits usually increase. The increased fat deposits vary from one patient to another and from one gender to another. Women tend to store more fat deposits in the hip and thigh areas where men tend to deposit fat in the abdominal area. These changes are most likely to occur in people after the age of 35 and are generally related to some hormonal changes (which you will read about later in this book) and dietary habits which promote the accumulation of fat tissue.

The skin, which is a wrap of the entire body, suffers as a result of years and years of exposure to environmental elements such as sunlight, radiation, weather, and trauma in general. In particular, the skin experiences significant wrinkling, broken veins, discoloration, rough texture, increased presence of skin moles, and hyperpigmented lesions.

Other things such as pregnancies, accidents, cuts, trauma, and bone diseases can affect the overall anatomy of the body.

It is important to understand the changes that occur on the body because those changes are directly related to the complaints that patients usually develop. Luckily, procedures have been developed to address the concerns and complaints of these problematic areas of the body.

Aging of the Neck

The way a person's neck ages depends on the gender as well as the body type of the individual. Basically, the aging of the neck takes on one of two forms.

TURKEY NECK

> **Telltale signs of a "Turkey Neck"**
>
> - Thin, damaged skin
> - Exhibits numerous broken veins
> - Several red and brown spots
> - Excessive skin that hangs

First of all, there is the classic "turkey neck", which is a neck that is very skinny and the muscle action over the skin is very severe. Usually the skin is quite thin and damaged. Typically there are many broken veins, brown and red spots, and many pigmentation problems. Because of the muscle action underneath, we usually see excessive hanging skin. There is a special muscle in the neck called the "platisma" which is generally responsible for the turkey neck appearance.

In the past, the primary treatment for the turkey neck condition has been the classic neck lift. However, this traditional procedure can be rather traumatic. It utilizes an incision that starts above the ear and goes around the hair and to the back of the head. This invasive treatment is done with general anesthesia or IV sedation and requires a significant amount of recovery time. This is because there is significant dissection and the detachment of the skin from the muscles can cause bleeding, scarring, infection, and other complications which can arise. If the patient can afford the massive amount of recovery time, this surgery offers tremendous results.

Because the majority of patients cannot endure the long recovery period of the classic neck lift, there have been recent attempts to perform a combination of noninvasive procedures to correct the problem of the turkey neck. Because the initial problem is caused by different factors at different levels, the treatment must be performed via multiple procedures. You simply cannot address a neck problem with one procedure.

Using a combination of procedures does offer the patient excellent results. Usually, in this type of treatment, we combine three procedures:

1)   Muscle control with the use of thread lifts

2)   Skin tightening

3)   Skin thickening, which is a process of skin restoration

Special treatments can also be included that enhance and increase the youthful appearance of the patient. For example, if there is undesirable hair, hair removal with IPL can be extremely beneficial. Removal of skin lesions and moles on the neck can also improve the overall health and appearance of the neck.

Although there is no down time, the process can be slow. The combination of multiple procedures can take as long as six months to a year to complete. Despite the extended period of time a patient has to wait to achieve their desired cosmetic effects, they tend to prefer the noninvasive procedures to the traditional methods.

Recently, newer surgical techniques have been developed and show promise for the future because only local anesthesia is used and the procedure is minimally invasive.

Newer thread lift procedures are becoming more popular and part of the cosmetic arsenal because they promise great results with minimal trauma and with local anesthesia.

Once again, the same principles that apply to the face also apply to the neck area. We need muscle control, lift, tightening, and skin repair.

SHORT NECK

Another common problem of the neck is often referred to as "short neck" or "fat neck." This is quite the opposite of the turkey neck problem. With the turkey neck, we see significant muscle action. With the short neck, the anatomy of the neck has changed so much that we cannot see the definition between the neckline and the hair.

This type of neck usually has good skin condition, but has some loose skin in the neck area. There are usually significant amounts of fat deposits and the anatomy of the neck area is somewhat deformed. The muscles seem to be almost detached from the neck area, which has resulted in a straight line from the face down to the chest. The loss of definition from the face to the chest has been the major complaint of patients suffering from this condition.

Treatments for this condition attempt to improve the anatomy, the curves, and the lines between the face and the neck. It's important to have good definition between the jaw line and the neck; otherwise the cosmetic appearance of the face is poor.

"Your body is a temple, but only if you treat it as one."

~Astrid Alauda

Although the skin condition of this type of neck is usually better than that of the turkey neck, the use of lasers, IPLs, and good skin repair are still important. Since there are some fat deposits, liposuction can help in some cases.

After removal of the fat and skin repair is performed, skin tightening should be done. In order to define the lines, a lift is essential. Either the traditional lift can be done or a modified mini-lift can be performed. A thread lift procedure can be used with excellent results to restore the contour and the lines of the neck, which give the patient a more youthful appearance.

Sometimes, a facelift must be done in order to improve the appearance of the neck. The neck lift alone may not give the desirable results because the skin needs to be pulled upwards and sideways to obtain a nice definition of the chin, jaw line, angle of the mandible, and the neckline.

Although the neck is one of the most difficult areas for treatment, it is the next most requested area for treatment after the face. Because of this high demand, we can expect new procedures to be developed. To complicate matters more, there is a huge variance of cases from the skinny turkey neck to the fat short neck. To accommodate these individual differences, treatments should be customized to a patient's specific needs.

Unfortunately, due to the anatomy of the neck and the high degree of motion, neck rejuvenation treatments have a short life regardless of which procedure was chosen. Significant maintenance and follow-up procedures should be done often to maintain desired results.

OTHER FACTORS AFFECTING APPEARANCE

Factors such as thyroid disease, obesity, some types of medications can affect the appearance of the neck. Treating the diseases can improve the appearance of the neck. Therefore, we always recommend evaluating the patient's overall health because health and beauty cannot be separated. You don't want to be blowing against the wind; that is treating the neck whose condition is being caused by a systemic disease. Usually diet and exercise will help to control the medical condition and will help to maintain the results of the cosmetic treatment of the neck.

Aging of the Chest

The aging of the chest is less remarkable in men, but more so in women due to the presence of the woman's breasts. The breasts of a woman probably undergo the most significant changes throughout the body because of changes that occur throughout a woman's life. Events such as puberty, pregnancy, hormonal changes, weight gain or loss, can all change the form of the breast.

Generally, there are two major breast complaints.

PTOSIS

With the first complaint, the breast tends to have atrophy. In this case, the patient complains of small, flat, and droopy breasts, which we refer to as "Ptosis." As with most conditions, there are different degrees of Ptosis. For different degrees of Ptosis, there are different degrees of treatment.

A Piece of History

The first surgical breast augmentation was performed in 1890 using paraffin injections. In 1920 this technique was abandoned in favor of fat transplants. Fatty tissue was surgically removed from the abdomen and buttocks and transferred into the breasts. In the 1950's polyvinyl "sacs" were frequently used to achieve fuller, more projected breasts. Although invented in the early 1960's, it wasn't until the 1980's that the silicone implant, as we know it, really began to take off.

BREAST HYPERTROPHY

Then we have the other group; the women who have larger and heavier breasts, which tend to drop. We refer to this as hypertrophy. Hypertrophy ranges from mild to gigantomastia. In severe cases of hypertrophy, breasts can sometimes equal as much as 20 to 30 percent of the overall body weight. Such large breasts often pose serious medical problems due to the excessive weight on the spine and neck.

Beauty by the Numbers

More than 2.5 million women in America have breast implants!!

TREATMENTS FOR THE AGING CHEST

Noninvasive treatments for the breast are yet to be well developed. There are no significant treatments or procedures that do not involve some form of surgery. Although commercials advertise special creams and bras, nothing has been proven to improve breasts.

There are devices out there with the idea to lift and tighten the breasts, but we have yet to find a device that really makes a difference.

Noninvasive procedures such as lasers, range of frequency and other tightening machines has not been shown to efficiently treat breast problems. At this time, the solution for the aging breast is still surgical. Nevertheless, surgery has improved considerably.

If you review the history of breast surgeries, it is absolutely amazing to see the progress that has been made. Breast surgery used to be a major operation-- very often with a skin graft, loss of sensitivity, loss of ability to breastfeed, blood transfusions, and general anesthesia. Breast surgery has gone from being a major undertaking to a comfortable procedure, which is less aggressive and less traumatic to the patient. Most of the breast procedures today are able to preserve the sensitivity around the nipple area. Although major improvements have been made, it is still surgery and requires some amount of recovery time and some form of general anesthesia or IV sedation.

Treatment of the Ptosis breast is the breast lift. There are several methods of performing the breast lift. The most common procedures tend to be ones with minimal scarring. For example, there is a scar that has the appearance of an inverted "T" with a vertical and horizontal incision.

Beauty by the Numbers

In 2007, 153,087 women had a breast reduction.

There is an "L" shaped scar, which avoids an incision on the inner part of the breast.

As mentioned before, the trend is to use procedures with the least amount of scarring. One of the biggest advantages in breast surgery is the use of breast implants. Although very controversial, breast implants are very popular.

Treating Hypertrophy of the Breast

The most common procedure to treat hypertrophy of the breast is breast reduction surgery. Before surgery, the surgeon will typically ask the patient to sit upright so that he or she can draw surgical markings upon the breast. The markings are to indicate the upright position of the breasts so that the proper incisions can be made during surgery while the patient is lying down.

During surgery, an incision is made along the surgical markings. Flaps are created on both sides of the breast and the excess skin, fat, and glandular tissues are extracted. In most cases the nipples are moved to a higher position on the breast, but remain attached to the nerves and blood vessels. For very large breasts, however, the nipples may need to be moved and grafted to a completely new location. In these cases, the nipples are removed from the underlying connecting tissues and sensation is often lost in the nipple and areola.

After surgery, the flaps of skin (that were once above the nipple) are refolded around and beneath the breast, pulled to the front of the breast around the nipple, and sutured in place. The reduction of breast tissue and skin reduces the weight of the breast and reshapes it into proportion.

Upon completion of the procedure, stitches remain around the areola and nipple area, in a vertical line beneath the nipple and horizontally under the breast. If the breasts were not too overly large, then some surgical techniques can avoid the horizontal scar altogether.

Final Advice

If you are unhappy with the appearance of your neck or breasts or some other part of your body, you could be an ideal candidate for cosmetic surgery of the body. However, it's important to remember that cosmetic surgery is meant for improvement, not perfection. Also, to make your cosmetic surgery experience as successful as possible, be sure to select a qualified cosmetic surgeon. Below are questions to ask when looking for a potential cosmetic or plastic surgeon:

- Are the desired results I described realistic?
- Where will the neck lift or breast surgery be performed and how long will it take?
- Which procedure(s) would be the most appropriate for improving the appearance of my body area (i.e. liposuction, neck lift, breast augmentation)?
- What kind of anesthesia will the surgeon use during the surgery?
- How much does this treatment cost and what other elements factor into that cost (i.e., hospital fee, anesthesia, etc)?
- What is the surgeon's level of experience in performing the desired procedure?
- What percentage of patients experience complications with this particular procedure?
- What is the surgeon's policy in regards to correcting or repeating the procedure if the surgery does not meet agreed upon goals?
- What should I expect, post-operatively, in terms of soreness, scaring, activity level and so on?
- Have you ever had your malpractice insurance coverage denied, revoked or suspended?

✎ Dr. De Souza's Secret ✎

Other professionals such as physical therapists, orthopedic surgeons can assist patients in optimizing their health. Even psychological evaluation may be needed in order to help the patient obtain optimal health status. The WHO defines health as 'a state of complete physical, mental, and social well-being and not merely the absence of disease or infirmity. Health is a cumulative state, to be promoted throughout life to ensure that the full benefits are enjoyed in later years. Good health is vital to maintain an acceptable quality of life in older individuals and to ensure continued contributions of older persons to society.

Just as you may want a youthful-looking face, you probably would like an attractive body. I can't say it enough—if you want to have a youthful face and body, you must be healthy!

> *"I know not what the future holds, but I know who holds the future."*
>
> ~Author Unknown

Chapter 9

Getting Ready for the Future

When the 21st century arrived, we received a huge inheritance of knowledge from the 20th century. More improvement was made in the areas of health and beauty than any other time period throughout history. We have begun this century with the capability of being able to transform lives. More than ever before, we can now control our destiny. We can feel good, live better, and live longer. For the first time, we can actually sit in the driver's seat and control what happens to our bodies.

"You'll only find what you're looking for, but you're only looking for what you know. And if you don't know, you won't find it."

It's now possible to break the taboo that says that our genes will determine the destiny of our health. The last two decades of the 20th century demonstrated without a doubt that our genes are in fact, not our destiny. Just because you think your genes are bad doesn't mean that you have to accept that. It's important to remember that some external environmental factors can essentially turn our genes on and off. This combination of turning genes on and off—known as "gene modulation"—can play a role in determining our appearance, our quality of life, and even the extension of our life. Knowing this allows us to have major control over our destiny.

During the last decade of the 20th century, new technology made great strides in improving the skin rejuvenation process. Although we have yet to fulfill the science fiction predictions made at the beginning of the century about how high-tech we would be at the end of the 20h century, we really can't complain. We may not yet have flying cars and cannot take vacations to the moon, but one thing is certain, we have seen a tremendous growth in technology, which helps us every day in almost every aspect of our life.

Helpful Hormones

We've learned that the interaction between our hormones, which pretty much acts as the conductor of the orchestra of our body, allows us to control the function and appearance of the body.

Every single cell and every single organ within our body is controlled by hormones. It's no surprise then that fluctuating hormones can disrupt functions of the body. Because we now have the knowledge and technology to change the quality and levels of hormones within the body, we can rejuvenate the body in both appearance and function. Despite the fact that we cannot turn back the hands of time, we can at least buy and optimize time.

Walking Through Medicine

The 21st century opened up a huge door, and it is up to us to take advantage of it. It's our responsibility as physicians and as patients to change the paradigm of health. The progress of medicine over the years has become very clear. We first started with the thinking that diseases had devil-like qualities and we didn't understand the nature of the disease. As soon as we learned diseases were not evil beasts lurking within our bodies, we came to the realization that maybe we can diagnose the disease. There's an old saying that goes, "You'll only find what you're looking for, but you're only looking for what you know. And if you don't know, you won't find it."

We took a big step toward medicine and health care as we know it today once we started to learn that disease is an organic process and could see the disease happening within our body. Through many years of research, doctors have been able to progress from simply knowing about diseases to treating diseases.

Did You Know?

Hormones are control chemicals that trigger major changes in the body. They control many important functions, including body chemistry, growth and sexual development, and the body's response to stress.

It's true that we finished the 20th century with a wealth of knowledge regarding the treatment of diseases, but that wasn't enough. Prevention became the next major trend. It was thought that if we could prevent the event from happening altogether, maybe we could have a better outcome. Now, thanks to innovations in medicine, we can find diseases early, treat them, and prevent them from becoming worse. While prevention was a wonderful step, this is still not the final step. The biggest step came at the very end of the 20th century and the beginning of the 21st century when we learned how to maintain health.

The primary goal of today's doctor should be to maintain health and not have to treat diseases as much as possible. Of course, eventually we do have to treat disease, because it's a fact of life. We also need to evaluate patients in the moment of death because death is a reality no matter how good medicine is.

The Changing Face of Plastic Surgery

The old classic concept of undergoing aggressive plastic surgery to make one major change on the face followed by seven days of hospitalization, plus weeks of painful recovery time is becoming a ghost of the past. Now patients have the opportunity to undergo a smoother procedure with several smaller procedures either done alone or in combination to produce good results without being profoundly noticeable and with minimal downtime. The idea is NOT to gain a youthful appearance in eighteen minutes but to gain eighteen years of your appearance in eighteen weeks with a number of small, smooth treatments that are barely noticeable by the people who are surrounding you at work or at home.

Beauty by the Numbers

According to the National Coalition on Health Care, nearly 90 million people - about one-third of the population below the age of 65 spent a portion of either 2006 or 2007 without health coverage.

A Piece of History

The Aesthetic Society, which has been collecting multi-specialty procedural statistics since 1997 says the overall number of cosmetic procedures has increased 457 percent since the collection of the statistics first began.

With the development of noninvasive plastic surgery procedures, nearly 11.7 million cosmetic surgical and nonsurgical procedures were performed in the United States in 2007, according to statistics released today by the American Society for Aesthetic Plastic Surgery.

Maintaining Health

All the studies and research clearly demonstrate that we will not be here forever and that the demise of the body is inevitable. However, we'd like to live as long as possible, look as good as possible, and get sick and die as fast and comfortably as possible.

As you've seen, 4000 years of history has moved us through some magical times. We went from not knowing what diseases are to learning what diseases are and how to help people with diseases, treat the disease, and eventually prevent the disease to now maintaining health.

This indeed, is not only a solution for health issues, but also for financial issues. It's much more cost effective to maintain health, then to treat a disease. The United States spends more than any other country in the world on health care. We spend about $1.3 trillion every year to treat disease. If we could do a better job maintaining health rather than treating diseases, we would only need to spend about one third of that amount on health care.

Financially speaking, maintaining health is a great concept and could be the key solution to reeling in our out of control healthcare system. We have over 40 million Americans without health insurance. Therefore, we must change things fast. We know what to do, and every segment of the society needs to mobilize to obtain what we call optimal health.

> **Opt3 Aspects of Patient Care**
>
> 1) Cosmetic Evaluation
>
> 2) Wellness Evaluation
>
> 3) Hormone Screening

The Optimal Health Institute Approach

We believe that the Optimal Health Institute approach is the future of healthcare. Patients will be seen in three major aspects. First of all, there is the cosmetic evaluation because everybody cares about their appearance.

The patient also needs to be evaluated for a sense of wellness. For example, what is their diet like, what is impacting them in their environment, what is their exercise regimen like? Over the years, patients' wellness aspect has been neglected by physicians and we're not sure why. Perhaps it's because they lack the knowledge. Personally, I must say that although I learned many great things in medical school, it didn't teach me enough about diet, nutrition, and exercise in order to teach someone.

And then it's essential to perform a screening to check hormone levels. As mentioned earlier, it's the hormones that control everything that happens within our bodies. If they are not in harmony, then our bodies will not be.

These three aspects need to be evaluated. Doctors such as plastic surgeons and cosmetic doctors, who have never approached wellness, fitness, anti-aging, will be forced to do it because their patients will not look good if they don't feel good, and they will not be pretty if they aren't healthy.

On the other side of the equation is the traditional physician--the same thing is going to happen to him or her. It won't matter if he is an endocrinologist, a cardiologist, or just your family physician because he too will also be forced to address issues related to your appearance because people want to look good — particularly when they feel good. If you wake up one morning and don't feel well, you may not even want to brush your teeth because you just don't care. But if you wake up in a good mood and are happy, you will want to look good and will want to get rid of some of the signs related to aging. Regardless of the patient's age, they will be asking the family physician, "What can I use on my face to look better? What should I use to protect my skin from the sun? What do I use for my nails and hair?" There will come a time when the physician will need to know this, but may not necessarily have to do all.

Final Advice

More and more clinics are joining forces to take a multidisciplinary approach when tackling anti-aging and wellness issues, but it doesn't have to get quite that complicated. This task can be accomplished in a simple fashion. The bottom line is that plastic and cosmetic surgeons need to be educated in health and the general physician needs to be educated about beauty. Because believe it or not, health and beauty unquestionably go together!! Furthermore, you will only succeed if you approach both at the same time. You cannot have true beauty if you are not healthy. That is the future and it shouldn't be a surprise. The real surprise is that the future is now and we are all looking for optimal health. And most of all what we want is for you to be a fabulously, beautiful, you!

🖎 Dr. De Souza's Secret 🖎

This is the time to take advantage of all the good medical breakthroughs from the 20th century. There are several very useful treatments in medicine to help you improve your appearance and your health such as vitamins, hormones, herbal and natural supplements as well as very good diets.

Keep in mind, however, the #1 rule for staying out of trouble. Never ever take anything without direction from your doctor, dietician or pharmacist. Using a natural vitamin can cause harm if it is not used correctly. Be careful but enjoy this large arsenal of new products just for you. If this book has taught you that time is not on your side, believe me, the technology is!!

Section II

Inner Beauty~ Anti-Aging Medicine Prof. Dr. Paul Ling Tai

CHAPTER 10

CHAPTER 10

New Beginnings!

"Life is not merely to be alive, but to be well."

~Marcus Valerius Martial

At the age of 63, I'm healthier and happier than I was at the age of 40!! However, it took traveling down many bumpy and treacherous roads to reach the point where I'm at in my life. For years, I thought I might not make it. You see, bad genes run in my family.

My family curse

My father and brother were both young when they died from heart failure. My dad was only 43 and my brother was 45. My second oldest brother had open-heart surgery when he was 42 and my mother has had two heart surgeries. Each one of these family members has always taken good care of themselves--none ever drank or smoked. Naturally, I was worried that I too, would someday fall victim to my family's genetic curse. But, recognizing that genetics are involved was my first step towards avoiding health problems that are known to run in my family.

Hello...time to wake up!!

Although I was deeply troubled by the deaths of my family members, the inherited health problems weren't enough to convince me to modify my lifestyle. I didn't change my way of living until I realized that I felt like the thousands of patients I've treated. It happened almost suddenly one day--I finally grasped what they were experiencing. I understood how they felt. I could actually feel their pain. Sure...I studied my patients' conditions. I examined them and later I treated them, but I never really knew how they felt until I felt the very same way. I finally woke up!!

From me to you

Throughout this book you will find amazing, yet practical adaptations of extensive medical research I've conducted and acquired throughout the years. This book is not intended for academic use, but rather for practical purposes. Through my own experiences and those of my patients, I will share with you ideas that work and those that don't. Every detail I share comes from the knowledge I gained from my years as a medical doctor as well as learning from all the wonderful doctors I've come to know and respect.

These chapters depict the story of my life, your life, and everybody else's life. It is the story of the complex organism we call the "*human body.*"

I didn't become a doctor just to earn a paycheck; I became a doctor so that I could learn how to save my own life. By writing this book and sharing this critical health information, I now hope to help you save your life. This is practical knowledge that will help to make you feel stronger, look younger and ultimately live longer.

How it all began

As a child, life certainly wasn't easy for me. But because I was exposed to the many trials and tribulations that people (including myself) around the world had to endure, I learned a lot about life—and people.

My father, who was a chemist, died from heart failure when I was only a year old. Needless to say, I never had the chance to know him. Shortly after losing my father, my younger brother died unexpectedly--he was only five-years-old.

A few years after my father died, my mother, a master acupuncturist and herbalist married a wealthy and kind Dutch import-export businessman. My stepfather was well known and well respected throughout Shanghai in the 1940s and 50s. Being the kind man that he was, he took in my siblings and myself and provided for us before communism took over.

Leaving China Behind

The Chinese government took everything he had away, which meant everything "we" had ended up in the hands of those who did not work for it. Communism overthrew capitalism and things started getting crazy in the city, which meant we needed to get out of China.

Being Chinese aristocrats had its blessings and its burdens. Our family was once respected, but during the shift in government we were cursed and spat on. Fortunately, my mother kept in touch with old friends. One of her friends happened to be the wife of a Brazilian ambassador so we took advantage of our connections and applied for visas. Months later, the Chinese government notified us that our whole family was allowed to leave China--unharmed.

For us to leave Red China in 1954 was like winning the lottery! And I sincerely mean that! Especially since I had a brother and sister who were of age to be in the "People's Army." During that time, Chinese communists wanted every able-bodied teenager for its military. I was only 7-years-old so I didn't have to worry about any of that stuff. I just followed my family around the world and into Brazil.

Did you know?

The Chinese Communist Party (CCP) is the world's largest political party. It had 72.39 million members in 2006, but these members only account for approximately roughly 5 percent of China's population.

Starting Over

Life in Brazil wasn't easy. We were forced to leave our home of comfort and luxury behind in China—forever! We were now strangers in a foreign land. We didn't speak the language, nor did we understand the culture. With no money and few friends, we depended on the Brazilian embassy for assistance. They gave us a tiny, closet-like apartment to live in along with a few occasional loaves of bread to eat.

When the little money we had ran out, my incredibly resourceful mother decided it was time to sell some of our belongings door-to-door.

Although dinner in Brazil was a rarity back then, my mother still made the family sit together every evening. She referred to these evening gatherings as "family meetings." Occasionally, we were able to have a few pieces of bread, or a can of sardines to munch on while we discussed the status of our current situation. During one particular family meeting, my mother asked my siblings (who were all older than I) to help her sell some of our family possessions, but they refused. I assumed they snubbed mother's request because asking strangers to buy *our* things was far too embarrassing an act for my "cool" teenage siblings to engage in. But I, being the youngest and most eager to explore, happily volunteered. I was thrilled, because helping my mother meant spending all day with her.

Life's Lessons

Together, Mother and I sold tablecloths, handkerchiefs, chopsticks, and small porcelain items. As we ventured through the back streets of Sao Paulo, not only did I learn Portuguese, I learned a lot about people.

One lesson I learned was that "People are naturally good and just as they have helped us, I want to help them." I believe if they are approached honestly and straightforwardly, people will more than likely help you, and if anyone needed help, we certainly did.

I became known as Sao Paulo's 7-year-old Chinese sales boy.

My mother, a beautiful and sincere woman, towered over me as I led the way through the alleys and back streets of Brazil speaking broken Portuguese and selling trinkets door-to-door. That is how I survived and that is how *we* survived.

Going to America

One day out of the blue when I was 17, my mother surprised me by telling me that I was to go to America. "How could I go to America?" I thought. After all, I finally had friends, a girlfriend (my first), and a great teenaged life. Despite my energetic protestations, I was unable to influence her; she was determined to send me to the United States and there wasn't anything I could do about it.

Everything seemed so surreal, like a bizarre dream. It didn't really hit me that I was leaving Brazil until I found myself at the airport with my bag in hand.

You may not know this well-guarded secret, but traditional Chinese families rarely, if ever touch one another. Hugs and kisses are never to be shared. The first time I ever had any physical contact with my mother was at the Sao Paulo Airport where she shook my hand as a gesture for goodbye. Moments after, she tightly rolled a crisp American $100 bill and placed it in my top-left shirt pocket. I read her eyes as they spoke to me and said, "Don't call me, I'll call you." Twelve years passed before I saw or spoke to my mother again. Until then, there were no telephone calls, letters or visitations.

Warm, compassionate hearts

Once in America, I became my best friend, caretaker and confidant. Yet, I was fortunate enough to have found a generous family in Oregon who sponsored me for eight months. It was there where I learned how to speak English and I learned how to act like an American. Many more kind-hearted American families adopted me along the way and fed me when I was really hungry and gave me shelter when I had nowhere to go.

Life gets busy

Upon finishing medical school, I sharpened my skills as a surgeon and a clinician during a hospital surgical residency in Detroit, Michigan. As I rotated throughout all the hospital departments, I found that I definitely enjoyed the emergency room best. I loved the drama, the adrenaline, and the blood and glory of the emergency room.

After working diligently for a few years, I was able to build one of the most successful reconstructive surgical clinics in the U.S. My specialty was foot, ankle, leg, bone, joint and tendon reconstruction. Between my partner and I, we saw over 100 patients each day. Our facilities, which were state-of-the-art, were equipped with our own internal radiology and physiotherapy departments along with an ambulatory surgical center.

Day after day, patients regularly complained of broken-down joints, and were plagued with health problems such as diabetes, arthritis, abnormal blood work, and deteriorated central and peripheral nervous systems. All I knew how to do was fix, patch, repair, and send them on their way. It wasn't until I turned 40 when I began to understand the underlying health problem of my patients. It's a little phenomenon people call "**aging**. "

"Aging is a high price to pay for maturity."

~Author Unknown

Aging isn't easy. In fact, it can drop a person to their knees. Everyday seems like torture. I know this firsthand as I once allowed myself to succumb. It took me almost six decades of living to realize that I needed to drastically change my lifestyle by starting at the roots, the core, and the base of what moves me. I became the patient and the physician and searched for a way to treat myself. After conducting extensive research, I realized the key to healthy living is having healthy, balanced hormones--**the natural way!!!!**

Feel better the natural way

Natural supplementation via bioidentical hormones has made my life and the life of my patients so much better. We no longer suffer from the crippling pain of inflammation. We no longer watch ourselves wither away in despair due to a lack of energy and sexual vitality. Nope...not anymore....thanks to all of the amazing health secrets I've uncovered through my years of practice and research.

My motivation for writing this book is to share with you my passion for health and personal power--the passion I feel every day!!

I'm certain that the information I've accumulated over the years as a physician will enrich your life so that you can enjoy the benefits of break-through anti-aging technology just as much as I have.

Long ago, I had a vision that started me on a life-long journey to find health the natural way. My endless hours of grueling research, hard work and perseverance have turned my dreams and visions into a reality. The results of my relentless quest lie within in these pages — *Fabulously Beautiful You*. I hope you enjoy these health secrets and most importantly, I hope that you practice them daily.

Have a blessed life and please take responsibility for your health so that you may be healthier, feel stronger, look younger and ultimately live longer!

CHAPTER 11

So just how old are you?

"We have a lot to do...People don't seem to understand this. They think we're sitting in rocking chairs, which isn't at all true. Why we don't even own a rocking chair!"

-Sadie Delany, 103, on her 101-year-old sister and herself

There are thousands of people in the world like the Delany sisters' who are alive and well into their early hundreds. Journalists who have hiked to mountainous regions in faraway places such as Ararat, Turkey, and Damavand, Iran have reported to have visited 115-year-old men and women. When asked how they've managed to stay alive for so long, despite tumultuous weather conditions and unpredictable harvests, these men and women said they owed it all too how they felt and how often they've kept busy.

The health and longevity of people throughout the world has been attributed to the blend of diet, climate, emotional well-being, stress and physical activity. Compared to how most Americans live, a mountaineer's living conditions would be considered well below the poverty level. Born in huts made of decayed vegetable matter found in bogs without the presence of doctors, mountaineers' birthdates are remembered by seasons.

Many "115 summers old" men and women have been said to show physical signs of attentiveness by responding when spoken to, laughing, talking and walking at a moderate pace. To people like the mountaineers of the Caucasus mountain range, age only matters if you're cheese.

So what about you? How old are you? I don't just mean how long have you been on this earth--but how old do you actually feel? There is a big difference between a person's chronological age and biological age.

"You're only as old as you feel"

How long have you existed?

First of all, it's important to establish that *chronological age* is the day and year of your birth date subtracted from today's date; it's used to determine exactly how many years you've existed. Chronological age cannot be controlled, it cannot be changed. If you were born in 1960 and it is 2008, you most definitely have existed for 48 years. Now *biological age* on the other hand, is a different sort of animal. It deals with the inner you and follows no rules. It doesn't say, "Well, if I was born in 1960, I must be 48." No, the inner you can be younger or older, depending on how you treat yourself, how your body ages, and how your hormones are produced.

As years go on, your health problems and appearance only get worse if you continue living a life chock-full of bad habits (e.g. sleep deprivation, high-carb diet, smoking, substance abuse, etc.) and if your hormones continue to diminish. Whoa! Wait a minute! Hormones? What do diminishing hormones have to do with growing old? Plenty…read on!!!

Keeping your body in check

Hormones act as balancers by helping to align how you feel with your chronological age. Thus, the balancers of the body must be kept steady or your body will not feel as beautiful and energetic as it should. If you want to feel younger and more beautiful, pay special attention to your hormones.

Hormones 101

Hormones are natural compounds produced by the body's glands (adrenals, thyroid, ovaries, etc.). All hormones are made from cholesterol and act as messengers or signals between the nervous system and vital organs such as the brain, heart, and lungs. Like teachers in a classroom, they maintain order and give instructions. They work to regulate bodily functions so you can go about your daily activities without much difficulty (e.g. eating, drinking, visiting the little girl's room, learning, remembering and getting physical — the desire to touch, have sex, or fight).

The word hormone originates from the Greek word meaning "to urge on." Holding true to its meaning, in order for a person to live and be active, they need hormones. As hormones flow into our bloodstreams they work throughout the entire body, inside every cell, nerve and organ. The glands that produce hormones are called endocrine glands, hence the word endocrinology, which is the study of hormones and considered to be one of the most complex fields in medicine.

Hormones are major parts of an extremely complex network of signals; they concentrate on specific tasks that prompt various kinds of biological responses, which is why they're referred to as "the movers" of the emotional and physical well-being. Virtually each one of our organs and tissues are affected by hormones. Hundreds of them concentrate specifically on the task they were meant to complete. When one or more of the hormones are deficient, other hormones must work harder to pick up their slack or the job does not get done! By doing this, their strengths become their weaknesses. In essence, hormones define us. They affect our personality and express our DNA; they can work with you or against you. Hormones form your whole being. Treat them well and they will treat you well!

Hormones are the good guys

Hormones are basically like friends who attempt to finish your sentences and tell you things you'd rather not know. Hormones help your body feel certain ways and can be activated in many different ways at different times of the day. You may not always be able communicate the sensations you experience verbally, but if you pay close attention to the feelings you're experiencing, you may be able to distinguish which hormone caused a particular signal, and how you communicated the signal through response.

Some hormone levels are higher in the morning (e.g. cortisol) getting you ready for a busy day with full energy, and some of them are higher in the evening (e.g. melatonin) getting you ready to go to bed, feeling sleepy and drowsy. Some hormones circulate when you are upset, pleased, or anxious, and they can be initiated through each of the five senses. Subsequently, your senses act as historians in that they register information sent by nerves and shoot chemicals to your brain from your hormones. How these feelings are expressed is completely up to the individual.

Listen To Your Body

Hormones can cause your body to say different things. An absence of certain hormones can cause tremors, twitching, irregular heartbeats, and an assortment of other internal disruptions that will make you act in ways that is difficult for you to control.

To a large extent, you are what your hormones are because they regulate everything. If you're to remember anything from this book, remember that your hormones regulate all internal functions. They're the body's administration and government — they're the police officers and message carriers. Hormones try to avoid chaos and keep the peace, and as faithful soldiers, they fight for you until their demise. When they are exhausted, the hormone production is minimal and you feel very, very old.

Hormones are released in response to various sorts of environmental and internal conditions so that you can adjust to various situations and surroundings. For example, because of hormones, we have depth perception, which prevents us from falling down stairs. Our hormones tell us when we need to take larger and longer steps, and by the same token, when we need to take smaller steps. If it weren't for our hormones, our bodies would be bruised and broken. Even though our eyes usually get the credit for keeping us moving in the right direction, it's really our hormones that deserve the recognition.

Open the Door to Your Health

Acting as a key, hormones roam around freely in the bloodstream, just waiting to be recognized by a receptor cell acting as a lock (these can only be activated or unlocked by a specific type of hormone) that will take them to their assigned destination. As a key is to a lock, once activated, the cell knows when to start a specific function for the body to perform.

The body contains more than 100 trillion cells and hormones are the chief regulators of these trillion and some cells. They control everything — including every heartbeat, breath and flexed muscle. By depositing and burning fat, hormones build strong bones and regulate metabolism, which controls heat and energy production. In addition, hormones define female and male characteristics associated with sexuality — where do you think the terms sexy and sex appeal come from?

Battle of the sexes (or hormones)

Although hormones affect both sexes' decision-making, memory and self-confidence, which in turn affect personality, character traits and behaviors, hormones do perform different functions for males and females.

Hormones control a woman's body by giving her a monthly menstrual cycle (allowing her to give birth) and lactating ability (for breast feeding). When and if a woman becomes pregnant, it's hormones that set the time for her to deliver the baby. These very same hormones give a woman's body the ability to cope with stress (which has potential to develop into depression), prevent fatigue, and provide a sense of calm during times of anxiety.

In men, hormones define their masculinity. Men are hairy because of their hormones. Men can develop muscle quicker than women because of their hormones. Men have a stronger sex drive because of their… you guessed it, hormones.

Let's get the party started!

I hope I've enlightened you just a bit about your hormones. I wanted to share the excitement with you over the importance of your hormones, particularly with regard to your physical responses and immunities. Like a climax in a movie, a story, or in the bedroom, hormones have their ups and downs. Your hormone levels are at their highest around the age of 20 to 25. After that, they start to diminish—slowly, gradually and consistently. Because of this, the immune system is weakened and the person experiencing a hormonal deficiency is more likely to experience difficulty fighting disease and infection, compared to a person who has replenished and functioning hormones.

A big, happy hormone family

As members of the endocrine system, glands manufacture hormones. Hormones are released by the thyroid, parathyroid, adrenal and other glands, under the general direction of pituitary gland, "the father." Glands work together in unison just as a family would.

Come on in and meet the family...

This is...

Hypothalamus: Mom, whom we love and know for the commands, 'Go ask your father' and 'Don't tell your father.' A central area on the underside of the brain that secretes hormones that stimulate or suppress the release of hormones to the pituitary gland.

Pituitary: Dad, who makes sure we have everything we need, all the time. Tough at times, he makes sure everything runs smoothly at home. The master gland secretes hormones that influence many other glands and organs, affecting growth and reproduction.

Pineal: The little brother that never wants to get up for school, a.k.a. 'Sleepy.' Secretes melatonin (promotes sleep), a hormone involved with daily biological rhythms.

Thyroid: The older sister that's always on the run. The family's chess club champion and theatrical diva. Located on the neck, regulates metabolism and blood calcium levels.

Adrenal: The cousin all your girlfriends want to date. He's 'The Fonz'. He's 'Mr. Cool,' both a lover and a fighter. Located above each kidney, they secrete cortisol as anti-inflammation, response to stress and androgens ("male" hormones) like cortisol, and aldosterone, which helps maintain the body's salt and potassium balances. Also stimulates T-cell development for the immune system and epinephrine (adrenaline) and norepinepherin (noradrenaline) which are involved in "fight or flight" responses.

Ovaries: The aunt, a feminist. She applauds anything a woman does, and is known for throwing "first time period parties." Secretes "female" hormones like estrogen for development and maintenance of female characteristics. Also secretes progesterone to prepare the uterus for pregnancy. Most importantly the ovaries produce eggs for fertilization.

Uterus: Grandma, she can be spotted doing laps around the neighborhood at 5 a.m. Secretes hormones and proteins that are almost always in response to the cyclical hormonal changes in a woman.

Testes: The hyperactive uncle, who's always giving everyone motivational speeches and pep talks, produces testosterone and sperm.

Pancreas: The motor-mouth cousin, niece or daughter who's always complaining about her weight. She's either too thin or too big. Nevertheless, she's a sweetie and is filled with energy. Secretes insulin; controls the use of sugar in the body and other hormones involved with sugar metabolism.

Nobody lives forever—including hormones!

Aging is nature's way of preparing us for death. Many of us will begin to lose appetite, yet we'll gain weight. We'll have trouble urinating, yet we feel urgency to go. Some of us will have to go more often than others, and some of us won't go as often as we should. The same applies for sleeping: Some of us will feel sleepy all the time, and others will feel sleepy and have trouble waking up. Hormone loss place such an enormous burdens on us that dying sooner may seem like a better idea than dying later.

When you complain about how "old" you feel, this means you're losing hormones. Next time a friend asks you how you're feeling, instead of saying not so great, tell him or her that your hormones are diminishing. Most likely, you'll get a peculiar look from them, but at the same time, perhaps it will give them "a heads up" should they ever experience similar problems.

Mirror, mirror on the wall

Our hormones reflect our age as a mirror reflects our image. Primary hormones are anabolic. Physicians and researchers use this term for something that supports life and to describe the cell activity that helps your body build cells and proteins that give thickness and quality to your skin and organs. There are also, of course, catabolic hormones, which take part in the normal process of breaking down protein and cells.

Between the ages of 20 and 25, the balance of anabolic processes (build-up) reaches its peak. After the age of 20, there's a slight possibility that the body may grow a tad bit more, but after the age 25, growth is highly unlikely. By this I mean, when we're young, our entire being is growing, getting taller, larger and our DNA is developing to its fullest at this stage we have a large net of positive anabolic hormones.

Between the ages of 30 and 35, the anabolic mechanism peaks and plateaus. Between 35 and 40, our anabolic hormones begin to stabilize. Thereafter, the balance of anabolic and catabolic starts to tilt slightly more toward catabolic. This means our bodies start to deteriorate in quality. The tissues and proteins in our organs dwindle away as our energy and vitality lessen more and more with time and hormone depletion.

> **STOP AND THINK**
>
> *Samuel is aging prematurely. What do you think will happen to him? Which diseases is he likely to contract from his lack of immunity and from his current cardiovascular system status? Are there ways to revive Samuel's hormones? What can be done to help Samuel look better? Does Samuel have to go on living this nightmare? Do we have to live like Samuel? The answer is NO!*

From this point forward, the net result is that we become slightly more catabolic than anabolic. From age 50 on, this catabolic balance shifts at a much more accelerated rate. As you will learn later, our bodies are affected in so many ways when our hormones go into a drastic free fall. We lose most of the constructive building effects of "good" anabolic hormones every day to catabolic hormones. Take a look at yourself in the mirror and you'll see increased anabolic depletion through the lines and age spots on your face. You don't need fancy lab tests or a doctor to tell you that "baby, you ain't what you used to be."

Sam's Story

> *27-year-old Samuel is studying to join the seminary. People refer to him as the "friendly giant." He's 6-foot-5, which is taller than most guys. This also means there's a lot of focus on his abdominal and chest area, since most people are at eye level with these two areas of his body. Samuel's weight has increasingly become problematic, so he's embarrassed that people maintain eye contact with these areas instead of centering on his face.*
>
> *Lacking muscle tone, Samuel looks effeminate. Not only does he speak in a soft voice, but he has wider hips and larger thighs than most guys do. A lot of people assume Samuel's sensitivity to be a part of his personality, but it's not. Over the years he's complained about being single and appearing overly sensitive because of how he articulates himself. Samuel drags his words and takes longer than a few moments to complete a thought.*
>
> *At 27, Samuel is at his prime. If anything, he should be bouncing off the walls with energy. How was he to be the future leader of a religious ministry without energy? That's like having a toothless dentist fix your teeth!*
>
> *His lack of energy drove him to bed early and most of the time he would miss class in the morning because he'd sleep in. The guy was obviously depressed and definitely not in the best shape. As for his diet, I'd watch him finish up a whole chocolate bar in one office sit-in. He told me he did this often. Once, he said, he finished a box of 50 chocolates in one hour. I asked how and why he would do such a thing to himself. He responded that he's become so depressed he resorts to food, usually in the form of sweets.*
>
> *A complete hormone panel was taken from Samuel, checking his progesterone, testosterone, estradiol and DHEA levels. His biomarkers revealed that he was closer to age 73 than 27.*

Samuel's story perfectly describes all of the disparities between chronological and biological aging. Samuel might as well have been born 50 years earlier! Chronologically he's 27, but biologically, he's closer to 80 than he is 30. You may have met someone like Samuel and have asked yourself "What's wrong with this picture?" or, "What's wrong with what I'm seeing? Why is this young person so haggard looking? They look so tired and so stressed when they're supposed to be at their prime!"

Now of course, we must be reasonable! We cannot expect a person who is 46 to look like they're 20, BUT they can look like they're 35 and feel like they're 20. The answer to this problem is to replenish our depleted hormone levels; however, many people don't use this knowledge to their advantage. Instead they take antidepressants, seek cosmetic surgery and spend thousands of dollars on facial creams that are packaged attractively and have pleasing scents, yet we haven't tackled the real aging problem. The mainstream of society is so used to trying to coat the problem and cover it up that they don't get to the heart of the real issue. We merely cover the problem like makeup covers up a pimple on a teenager's face.

What to do?

If you think your hormones are diminishing, there is hope!!! Allow a professional to evaluate your current hormone status, and amazing changes will occur if you follow your physician's directions. He or she will probably advise you to modify your diet and exercise plans and they will provide you with instructions for vitamin, mineral, and bioidentical hormone supplementations.

"Many people grow old before their time, but you don't have to!"

Bioidentical hormones

When I use the term bioidentical hormones, I mean natural hormones, not synthetic. So, what's the difference between the two? First of all, they're a world apart in how they affect the body. To avoid stating the obvious, bioidentical—or natural hormones—are 100 percent compatible with your body. Synthetic hormones, on the other hand, are often only six to eight percent compatible with your body. If over 90 percent of a synthetic hormone is incompatible with your body, severe side effects which cause irreversible damage to your body and health may result. Bioidentical hormones can be used through liposome technology, which can be rubbed, spritzed (sublingually), or even inserted (by means of suppositories).

Dispelling the myths

- **Do synthetic hormones work quicker?**

In almost every instance involving our present health care system, synthetic hormones are chosen over bioidentical hormones because of prescriptive or insurance reasons. Sadly, synthetic hormones have become the first choice because many people have been brainwashed into thinking that synthetic hormones deliver rapid results to problems that have worsened with time. This may be true, but then so is the adage "what begins too soon, ends too soon."

- **Do natural hormones make my glands sluggish?**

A common myth surrounding natural hormone replacement is that it can cause your own endocrine glands to become sluggish to the point that they eventually break down. This is false! It just isn't so. When your body's glands stop making a hormone or decrease the production of a particular hormone because they are "too tired" to produce any more of the hormones they're accustomed to producing, natural supplement hormones assist them in making the hormones your body needs. It actually gives them a "break" and "a lending hand." We all appreciate that when we are tired, don't we?

Endocrine gland exhaustion is a vicious cycle. The lower the level of hormones, the worse exhaustion can be for glands. The more your body demands hormones and doesn't get them, the more pressure is placed on those very same glands to produce when they're already exhausted and incapable of production. This increases stress, fatiguing glands and making them more likely to never produce hormones again.

You can't make a gland work any faster or any better than what your body's own mechanism of stimulation already has in effect. Every gland and every hormone has a chemical compound produced by the brain called a secretagogues, or a stimulating hormone, which prompts a particular gland to produce the hormone your body requires. Its natures already perfect balance.

If that stimulating hormone is not capable of making the target gland produce more of the hormone, it's because that gland is too tired and overworked to do so. When this occurs, no matter how many artificial stimulants you feed your gland, it's unable to produce any more hormones. In fact, forced continued stimulation has the tendency to only worsen matters.

Why our hormone levels decrease:

- Severe illness
- A history of major surgery or surgeries
- Internal aging (in other words, self-neglect)
- Depression
- A lack of exercise
- Insufficient amounts of sleep
- Increased stress levels
- Poor nutrition

Since hormones depend on each other to get various jobs done, if one collapses, the others must work more intensely to make up for its absence. If a hormone or a set of hormones work harder, the areas they were meant to serve will be neglected. One reaction triggers another—without one, you don't have the other, and eventually a person will suffer by becoming ill or appearing ill.

Is old age beautiful?

The United States is among the few countries in the world where age isn't regarded as being attractive. The "old" in America aren't graceful, nor are they beautiful. However, in countries like France and Italy, age is *sexy*. The difference between Americans and their Western counterparts are lifestyle and diet. An average day for an American consists of: working eight to ten hours; having a carbo-packed breakfast, lunch and dinner comprised of super-sized fast-food and refined sugars found in doughnuts, pastries, cake, smoothies, juices and sodas; and not exercising at all, or exercising too much.

Carbs that are consumed too often and too quickly will lead to higher cortisol levels, which can increase the pressures of stress even when stress isn't present. When the body triggers "high tension," the desire to eat is than increased by ten-fold; this leads into insomnia and obesity. Poor nutrition, fatigue, stress and a lack of sleep will destroy a person's hormones by exhausting the glands that produce vital hormones.

The last thing people want to do when they are tired is exercise. Speaking for myself, when I'm tired I feel like I'm strapped to a metal ball and chains. Muscles need to be put in use before they can build aerobic capacity, and how will that be possible for you to do if you're exerting all the energy you have by attempting to stay awake? This is neither possible nor expected.

Biological signs of aging:

- Lack of energy

- Being overweight
- Lagging libido
- Nervousness/ shakiness
- Fatigue
- Skin lesions/ wrinkles, sun spots, sagging skin etc.
- Variable appetite
- Poor memory
- Digestive problems/ frequent diarrhea or irritable bowel syndrome/constipation
- Sore joints
- Chronic pain
- Sleep problems
- Frequent allergies
- Low immunity

Implementing a bioidentical hormone plan can help reverse the aging process within your body, so you look as young as you feel.

So once again, how old are you?

Try to determine how old you are by recognizing where most of your health ailments are coming from.

- Can I remember things easily?
- Can I recall names of people, places, memories, etc?
- How often do I write notes to myself?

Ask yourself…

- How's my vision?
- How's my depth perception?
- Have I become clumsier?
- How's my hearing?
- How many times do I have to ask

And be honest about this…I mostly complain about…

- joint pain
- muscle pain
- headaches
- trouble breathing
- chest pains
- uneasy stomach
- constipation
- lax bowel movements
- hair loss
- feeling lethargic (weary)
- negative change in attitude
- increased wrinkles

🔖 Dr. Tai's Beauty Secret 🔖

In order to spare glands from severe fatigue, start your anti-aging bioidentical hormone replacement as soon as you notice symptoms of hormone depletion. Don't wait until you're totally depleted before starting replacement with natural bioidentical hormones. By then, it may be too late for you to start bioidentical hormone treatment because your glands have almost withered away. I can't stress enough the importance of replenishing hormones early.

In the future, don't be too surprised if we start to see bioidentical hormone replacement being used by people as young as 30. The environment is growing increasingly polluted, and demands are ever-increasing as the economy seems to be skyrocketing with technological advancements. Life is going to hectic for a lot of people and it'll only get more complicated. This can only mean that stress levels and blood pressures will go up with everything else.

This is why it would've been a smarter decision on our parts to have tested our hormone levels at the peak of our youth, instead of our clinging moments of desperation. However, we have not the time for regrets. Now is the time to do what you can! Intrinsic hormone abnormalities cause cravings for sugar and causes deficiencies in the metabolism such as hypothyroidism and DHEA scarcity. When hormone levels drop, you will begin to see an increase in weight gain (usually around the abdomen), which correlates with cardiovascular disease.

Find out how your body works and what it can and cannot handle. Natural hormones don't cause cancer, weight gain or heart disease. These side effects for hormone replacement are applied mostly to synthetic hormones only. There's been no researched evidence linking bioidentical hormones and diseases. However, an excess of anything can never be good, even in nature. Whether it be hormones, oxygen or water, too much of anything can eventually cause harm, just be careful and stick with the safest choices. You won't be sorry!

CHAPTER 12

Saliva Testing

"In order to change we must be sick and tired of being sick and tired."

~Author Unknown

I t's no secret that you are aging--your mirror will be the first to tell you. This means some of your hormones have gone missing in action, so the question you have to answer is-- which hormones? The first and most important step of bioidentical hormone treatment is determining your hormone levels. But what is the best way to accomplish this?

There are several tests on the market that can measure your hormones, but each comes with its own set of pros and cons. Through extensive research and laboratory trials, I've come to the realization that saliva hormone testing is by far the simplest and most accurate method for determining metabolic factors and biological age. With the help of a trained physician or expert health worker, you'll learn how to achieve and maintain a biohormone balance. Needless to say, no one should begin using supplements without first understanding how to balance them. Using bioidentical hormone supplements without an expert guiding you will not only prohibit you from achieving optimal results, it can also cause negative side effects. Only a trained expert can customize a life-long natural supplement plan tailored to you and only you.

> **Important terms to know:**
>
> **Free hormones:** Unbound by protein; ready to be used. These hormones are functioning, alive and active.
>
> **Bound hormones:** Inactive and unusable hormones.

Using your mouth wisely

While one can utilize a urine or blood test to determine their hormone count, saliva hormone testing is the easiest test in which you can directly and accurately measure "free unbound active hormones." Unlike hormones found in blood and urine, hormones found in saliva are free and unbound by protein and ready to be used by your body. This means saliva analyses can reflect the exact markers of your own working hormonal activity.

Free vs. unbound hormones

Hormones circulate throughout our bloodstream in the form of *bound* and *unbound* hormones. The bound hormone fraction is a biologically inactive hormone that is connected to albumin, cortisol-bound globulins (CBG) and sex hormone binding globulins (SHBG). These bound hormones make up to 99 percent of the total hormones that circulate throughout our bloodstream. Therefore, measuring hormones in our blood would reflect an extremely large number of inactive hormones – rather than active ones. What this means is that in order to achieve an accurate hormone report, multiple blood drawing attempts would be required. Most people hate getting poked once – who wants to subject themselves to that more than once?

Now on the other hand, unbound by any other protein, albumin, or globulin, "free hormones" make up a rather small fraction of hormones that circulate throughout a person's body. Free hormones are completely available for immediate use by organ and tissue receptors for the maintenance of the body's activity.

These small yet essential portions of free hormones represent only 1 to 5 percent of the total concentration of hormones in our blood, whereas in the saliva, free hormones are present 100 percent. Therefore, saliva testing is the most accurate and painless way to obtain a correct hormonal status report. Affordable and convenient, saliva samples are collected by spitting into capsule-sized tubes. They're then sent to laboratories for evaluation. Within days, the patient's physician is contacted with the results on free hormone (active and useable) count.

The truth is in your saliva

The ratio between saliva and hormones is always constant and interactive. For example, in a blood test, testosterone shows up as 100 to 1 (100:1). This means blood shows 100 times more testosterone than saliva would ever show.

Complicated when contaminated

Hormone counts will be inaccurate if the saliva becomes tainted due to bleeding gums or food contaminations. In a clinical study conducted to show the effects of food and drink consumption while testing progesterone levels, test results were altered measurably before and after a patient consumed milk. These results prove just how much eating and drinking can affect hormone levels.

Avoid contamination

Inaccuracy can be controlled by not drinking or eating two hours before testing. Other causes of saliva contamination could be due to a blood-related problem, which can often be difficult to detect. In hormone levels, blood exceeds the saliva by 50-100 times. For those whose gums bleed often, special attention should be given to avoid contaminating the saliva testing sample with blood.

Research has determined that blood contamination is visible to the naked eye when it approaches 0.156 percent. Its equivalent laboratory testing of the containment of blood at 0.156 percent contributes to approximately 3 to 7 percent of the total hormones being evaluated. Generally, this is the acceptable cut off rate for blood contamination in blood sampling, making it a laboratory technician's duty to reject any saliva samples contaminated by the slightest amount of blood.

Blood contamination can also be prevented by avoiding brushing and flossing your teeth two hours before samples are collected.

Pros and cons of saliva hormone testing

Studies on saliva testing are finally becoming more abundant as it becomes a more widely accepted practice. From the pharmacokinetic perspective, there is a lack of published information involving the medical phenomena involving various types and ranges of salivary delivery systems (i.e., transdermal hormone delivery shows an enhanced salivary presence).

The saliva sample collection poses minimal disturbance to the patient's lifestyle. These collections can be taken under any circumstance and are suggested to be taken during various concurrent symptoms, e.g. during stress attack episodes, weakness, dizzy spells, and before and after intense physical activities like playing sports. Saliva testing is simpler, convenient, non-evasive and much more appealing. It doesn't require a professional to draw blood because if you can spit, we can test.

Saliva testing is easy, convenient, and poses minimal disturbance to the patient's lifestyle.

What's normal and what isn't?

The specific timing correlations of hormone release give the patient and the physician a unique perspective on the pathodynamics of disorders, diseases, or perhaps normal, physiological functions that were unable to have been detected in previous examinations. This innovative approach to testing will open a brand-new horizon in our current knowledge of daily circadian cycles of biohormones.

Saliva hormone testing allows for multiple sampling collections to be taken throughout the day, thereby making it possible to get extremely accurate reliability assessments of hormone concentration, in spite of diurnal fluctuations.

Changing hormones

Some hormones go through long-term fluctuations, such as monthly profile fluctuations of estrogen and progesterone. For seasonal variations, in the summer, because of longer daylight hours, the body's testosterone reaches its highest peak, as opposed to the winter when the days are shorter. The difference in light affects certain hormones, i.e. melatonin, hence creating different levels of mood swings and sleeping patterns.

Practical experience has proven that randomly taken single collection blood or saliva hormone samples will present false and erroneous results. This is why it's highly imperative for a collection to have more than five saliva samples taken during different times of the same day. To avoid erroneous results, saliva should be taken exactly one hour after waking in the morning and every three hours thereafter.

Because hormones are produced in spurts every two hours, collecting saliva at various times of the day has the ability to determine the highs and lows of your hormones. For example, the hormone *testosterone* is higher in the morning than it is in the evening. *Cortisol* is also higher in the morning than it is in the evening. You see it's important that you not rely on a single random sample to evaluate your hormonal status. By taking five saliva samples (a sample every three hours throughout the day), your statistical chances of obtaining accurate hormone results are 87 percent higher.

Saliva hormone testing allows for specific hormones to be tested. It isn't a calculated sample, but rather a direct quantitative measurement of active free fraction hormones without the interference of bound hormones.

Saliva collection process

The sample collection process is non-invasive, painless and convenient. The

Precautions:

- If you're experiencing oral bleeding your saliva test will be rejected once it's reached the laboratory. Therefore, avoid taking the test if you're aware of the slightest possibility that saliva may be contaminated with blood.

- Discontinue hormone supplementation for 24 hours prior to collecting saliva samples.

- Don't eat, drink, or smoke an hour before each saliva sample collection. Water is fine; however, anything else poses a problem with regard to testing accuracy.

- Also, many people send in their saliva samples with ice packs. No ice packs are necessary.

procedure allows the laboratory to evaluate a mixed saliva sample from multiple collections to get an actual value of hormones with distinct diurnal fluctuations.

Whether you're measuring one hormone, or many hormones, five collection samples must be taken throughout the day to obtain the most accurate test results. When testing saliva you will be provided with special plastic, non-recyclable vials.

Each vial will come with a plastic straw to spit into, and a pack of labels to record your name, date and time when each saliva test was taken. Because hormones fluctuate it is extremely important to document each saliva sample with the exact time. In other words, the timing must be precise-- no approximations or guesstimates are allowed!

On label write:

- Date of collection: month, day and year
- Time of collection: hour and minute(s)
- The most obvious--your name. You'd be surprised how many people forget to write their name.

Directions for collecting saliva samples:

1. Precisely one hour after you wake up, take your first saliva test. Reach for your first vial-- spit, label and set aside. *There's no need to refrigerate, it's advised to keep vials at room temperature (70- F).*

2. The second saliva sample should be taken three hours after your first collection was taken. Do the same: spit, label and set aside. When spitting, use the straw as a suction device. Place tiny straw against tongue, draw saliva from tongue and eject into straw. You can't reuse a straw, as soon as one is used, throw it away.

   Saliva must fill at least half the vial. Cap the tube tightly after filling to avoid leakage.

3. You will need to do this three more times throughout the day, totaling five collections. Each collection must be, again, exactly three hours apart from each other.

Saliva samples should be sent for testing as soon as possible, but definitely within 2-3 days.

Saliva testing vs. other methods

By comparison, saliva hormone testing is relatively newer than serum and urine testing, yet it's been gaining momentum and acceptance because of powerful appeal, practical usage and simplicity. Only 25 years old, its presence in mainstream medicine has had a considerably lesser amount of published information on its clinical usage than that of blood and urine hormone testing.

Alternative Hormonal Testing Methods

Urine Testing:
A urine test is conducted by urinating into a special urine container. Urine tests measure clarity, odor, color, pH levels, protein, glucose and ketones to reveal clues to various conditions.

Pros:
- Urine can easily measure estrone(E1), estradiol (E2), estriol (E3), DHEA and metabolites, testosterone, pregnenonlone, progesterone metabolites
- Relative cost: $250
- 24-hour collection makes timing re: hormone dose less critical

Cons:
- Urine samples must be collected throughout the day. Urine sampling calls for 24-hour collection, making it inconvenient and disastrous.
- 3 – 4 weeks to get results
- Fewer labs available to run tests

Serum Testing:
Blood is drawn from the veins using a needle and syringe. Blood tests are done to obtain cells and extra-cellular fluid from the body to check its health.

Pros:
- Readily available, short turnaround time on results
- In use for a long time
- Relatively standardized results

Cons:
- Provides information on hormone level only during the moments blood is drawn
- Can be expensive
- Bound vs. free are calculated, not directly measured. May be inaccurate depending on SHBG levels
- Drawing blood is painful causing false (higher) levels of cortisol (stress hormone) due to the pain that the patient endures
- Does not take into account the hourly fluctuations of hormones
- Blood must be drawn at the laboratory by a professional health care worker

Cotton Salivates:
Requires patients to salivate on a cotton roll that is wrapped around a plastic retainer.

Pros:
- Especially convenient for children (below age 5), older patients (80+) and patients with specific abnormalities, as string on cotton rod serves as a choking preventative.

Cons:
- "The use of cotton salivates resulted in erroneous cortisol values." –*according to the investigative report of Dr. Garrence Trier (2004, June)*
- Garrence found that cotton substances are able to interact with cortisol by creating an affinity binding. In conclusion, it's best to avoid using these cotton devices in saliva hormone sample collection.

CHAPTER 13

Synthetic vs. Bioidentical Hormones: What's the Difference?

"That which is striking and beautiful is not always good, but that which is good is always beautiful."

~Ninon de L'Enclos

Like many people, I've been fooled many a times by the dazzling likeness of cubic zirconias and diamonds. While I can't tell the difference, unfortunately, my wife can. She has an exceptionally keen eye.

To the untrained eye (such as mine), a cubic zirconia (CZ) appears to be identical to a diamond. But it doesn't take a gemologist or a jeweler to note the main difference between high-priced diamonds and CZs--one is real, and the other... isn't. Synthetic hormones may look like it, but they do not function like bioidentical hormones.

So........

Just as deep mines make diamonds, your body makes hormones. Bioidentical hormones are made from the same compounds that produce hormones in your body (bioidentical literally means "identical to your biology"). Bioidentical hormones should not be confused with phytohormones, which are at times, combined formulations of herbal extractions and chemical substances. At other times, labels that read "phytohormones" are oral supplements that possess the ability to support the bioidentical hormone that you may be lacking. Bioidentical hormones work differently—they give you what you need, when you need it, without hardly any side effects.

> **Pop Quiz**
>
> **Fake or real: Which would you prefer?**
>
> - Monopoly money or *real, cold cash*
> - Plastic flowers or *real flowers*
> - Silicon breasts or *real breasts*
> - Acrylic sweaters or *cashmere sweaters*
> - Synthetic or *bioidentical hormones*

Unlocking the doors of the body

To help you visualize how natural hormones work, think about the way keys and locks work together. Specific hormone molecules are like specific keys — only one key (hormone) matches one lock (hormone receptor site). Just as a particular key is needed to open a door, a particular hormone is needed for your body to function properly. When a hormone and a receptor properly correspond with each other, they set off a chain of events that allows you to go on with your life, normally, healthfully, and functioning perfectly.

Potential side effects of synthetic hormones
• **Weight gain**
• **Depression**
• **Various forms of cancer**
• **Hormonal imbalances**
• **Memory loss**
• **Disease**
• **Loss of mobility**
• **Loss of libido**

Not the real deal

Phytohormones, or plant extracts, aren't identical to your body's hormones. The hormones found in plants such as red clover and black cohosh have to be converted inside your body by mixing with stomach acids and going through a sequence of chemical digestion before they can mimic your hormones.

Most plant extracts (phytohormones) work on keeping cell receptor sites busy so that the body's tissues require less hormone production. Bioidentical hormones replenish lost hormones while fortifying already existing hormones. Bioidentical hormone supplements support specific hormones that you may lack or have an excess of. (For example, for an estrogen excess, take bioidentical progesterone. For a testosterone deficiency, take bioidentical testosterone.)

Faster, but dangerous

Because the FDA considers bioidentical hormones to be natural regardless of their source, they cannot be patented. Synthetic hormones, or pharmaceutically produced hormones are created by drug companies so they can maintain a patent for particular drugs.

After all, there's big money in pharmaceutical drugs; it is a multi-billion dollar industry. People tend to favor chemicals because they think that chemicals deliver faster results. As a result, the big pharmaceutical companies put large amounts of money into research and development for a chemical and even more money marketing these products.

I agree that synthetic hormones do bring about rapid results, BUT they bring about rapid results with dangerous long-term effects. When you use synthetic hormones, you run the risk of damaging some parts of your body in order to fix another part. Is this really what you want?

In a nutshell, pharmaceutical companies can't patent drugs made from the same molecular structures as the kind found in your body. They make synthetic drugs look similar to your hormones but the body reacts very differently with negative side effects, as shown in countless in-depth published researches.

> **Dr. Tai's *something to think about*:**
>
> Would you feed yourself a similar substance you'd feed your car?

Synthetic hormones—more than meet the eye

> **Pop Quiz #2**
>
> Synthetic hormones are made from…
>
> A) Coal tar
> B) Horse urine
> C) Chemicals that will potentially cause cancer
> D) All of the above
>
> *Correct answer: D, all of the above*

The so-called "estrogen equivalents" sold annually to millions of women across the world are made from the urine of pregnant horses. And horses' estrogen is 200 times stronger than natural estrogens (Collins, J., What's Your Menopause Type. Roseville, CA: Prima Health 2000).

Synthetic hormones are created in laboratories and are mostly made from hydrocarbons, more commonly referred to as coal and tar derivatives. Among the hundreds of kinds of synthetic forms of hormones readily available, the attempted reproduction of testosterone, methyl testosterone, is made of ammonium ions. Truth be told, when in an alcohol form, methyl can be used as an industrial solvent, sort of like antifreeze. Chemically manufactured, methyl testosterone is nowhere near a reproduction of natural testosterone. Synthetic hormones like methyl testosterone and estrogen are multifaceted—they're complex formulas that can have a number of negative side effects on your body. Our bodies sometimes have difficulty filtering and processing complex forms of drugs. Conjugated estrogens like pregnant horse urine mixtures have approximately 30 different forms of estrogens, which only animal bodies can make the most of. Human bodies, which are much more complex organisms, can experience difficulty adjusting to derivatives Mother Nature intended only four-legged creatures with hide or fur to possess. I'm convinced that synthetic hormones aren't safe, yet somehow they've been approved by the FDA.

Quick Facts

* Premarin made from horse's estrogens, equilin and equilenin can cause side effects such as burning on urination, allergies, joint aches, and pains. *Ahlgrimm, M., The HRT Solution. 1999; New York: Avery Pub.*

* Synthetic Estrogen is not compatible to your body's estrogen receptors. *Sinatra, S., Heart Sense for Women. Washington DC; Lifeline Press, 2000.*

It's in the proof

During the past several years, millions of people taking synthetic hormones have said that their bodies started to go haywire within a matter of months; their *regular* internal functions became *irregular*. This doesn't surprise me — just like my key and lock example, synthetic hormones are very similar to the hormones our bodies produce. However, our body rejects the remaining amount that isn't similar.

The body exerts a great deal of internal power while trying to metabolize substances it can't recognize, resulting in irreversible long term damage we've clinically determined to have limited knowledge of.

In 2002, a study was conducted on healthy (free of life-threatening illnesses) post-menopausal women examining the risks and benefits of synthetic estrogen and progesterone. During the trial, 26 percent of the study's participants who used synthetic estrogen and progesterone were at risk of developing breast cancer. (Women's Health Initiative research team. "Risks and benefits of estrogen and progesterone in healthy post-menopausal women." *Journal of the American Medical Association*, 2002; 288:321-333.)

Bioidentical hormones

Active extractions from natural sources like soy beans and yams are good sources of bioidentical hormone. These extractions are identical in molecular structure to that of human hormones. If monitored, side effects of any kind are rare and uncommon.

Many doctors are now making the switch from synthetic hormone therapy to natural hormone therapy. This is because research has defined the lines between synthetic and natural hormone replacement.

Regardless of what medical trends appear to be, you ultimately do have a choice. It's your body and your decision, but before you do, allow me to ask a rhetorical question — would you choose a cubic zirconium over a diamond?

Powerful Reasons to consider Natural Hormones

1. Relieves symptoms
2. Prevents memory loss
3. Improves heart health
4. Prevents osteoporosis
5. Increases cell repair and growth

> **Did you know?**
>
> Estrogens derived from horses urine may stay in your body up to 13 weeks, in contrast to your natural estradiol which are eliminated from your body within a few hours. *Ahlgrimm, M., The HRT Solution. 1999; New York: Avery Pub.*

> **Beauty by the Numbers**
>
> Hormones derived from animals are 200 percent more potent than necessary, which can cause the body to act in very aggressive ways, e.g. developing certain forms of cancers, strokes and thrombophlebitis (blood clots).

Dr. Neal Rouser, author of *Natural Hormone Replacement for Men and Women: How to Achieve Healthy Aging*, commented on the Women's Health Initiative (WHI) (one of the largest and longest-running studies America has experienced thus far). Dr. Rouser said synthetic estrogens pose dangers women should pay heed to.

"In my practice of prescribing natural hormones to women for five years, I have never seen the problems and side effects as we have seen with synthetic hormones. Why not replace the body with naturally biologically identical hormones? Anything besides natural hormones, as we have seen with the recent discontinuation of WHI (Women's Health Initiative) trials is dangerous to a woman's health."

-Dr. Rouser

Okay, now what?

Thus far, you've learned how to figure out which hormones your body may be lacking and the difference between bioidentical and synthetic hormones. So now what? How do you get these missing hormones back into your body?

My philosophy has always been taking care of yourself should be a pleasure, not a pain. Hormone delivery is just as important as the hormone itself, because it's all about how it gets where it needs to be and when the hormone actually arrives at its intended destination. It's like when you go off on a trip, whether personal or business—the important thing is that you're going. Great! But how? How will you go? Will you travel by train, plane or car? Will you walk? Will you ride your bike? Can you afford a plane ticket, or is it more cost-efficient if you drive? So, if you drive, will you get there on time? You see, all of these things matter, and just as important as it is for you to get where you need to be, it's just as important for your hormones to do the same (if not more). Without your hormones, the only place you'll be is in bed, and we don't want that, do we?

Hormone Delivery

It was once thought that hormones could be delivered only through injection; fortunately, that's not the case today. Bioidentical hormones can be administered in a variety of ways and there are enough choices to make anyone spin their heads a few times. Nowadays, these methods include injections, dermal patches, gels, lotion, pills, tablets, rings and sprays.

As I'm certain you'll notice, I prefer more painless methods like sublingual sprays and transdermal liposome creams.

Injections

Besides being inconvenient, costly, time-consuming, and literally a pain in the butt, injections can give you more of a dosage than you actually need.

Injections	
PROS	**CONS**
• Fast delivery • Direct administration to blood • Sometimes, if you're lucky, you'll get a cool plastic bandage.	• Painful • Appointments are necessary • Expensive- (require weekly/monthly office visitations payment with added charge for substance in syringe) • Time-consuming • Dosages may be too high for person's physiological build

Injections can cause a specific hormone level to be higher than your body can tolerate. Moments after an injection, hormone levels can shoot up to several hundred percent beyond your natural optimum level, which means that receiving an injection would be like eating three meals in one hour when you're supposed eat three meals over the course of 12 hours. You may react differently, but most likely you'd get sick from indigestion. The same example can be applied to bioidentical hormonal injection. From subnormal, you've reached levels that exceed normal, and this abrupt change can upset your body.

Dermal patches

Transdermal patches are like stickers. The skin is waterproof; however, it's not oil-proof. Dermal patches use skin-compatible oily material that can pass through the skin's top-layer, the epidermis, making its way through the skin's sub-layer, the dermis.

As you can see in the table below, the cons of dermal patches are much less than that of injections. Even so, I find dermal patches to be just as inconvenient. By and large, dermal patches are used for patients who are lacking testosterone and estrogen (two hormones that can be attributed for masculine and feminine characteristics); dermal patches aren't commonly used for other forms of hormone therapy. They're rare, and you have to keep track of changing patches on a regular basis. Hormone patches are very similar to nicotine patches—for those of you that have tried to quit smoking, hormone patches are just like that, sticky backings that require daily attention.

Dermal Patches	
PROS	**CONS**
• Fast delivery • Direct administration to blood	• Painful • Limited hormone selection available in patch collection • Expensive • No cool bandage; patches aren't as cute.

Gels and lotions

As a form of hormone delivery, topical solutions have become increasingly popular. They're painless and yield effective results. All you have to do is pump, rub, hold off for a few moments before getting dressed, and out the door you go. I prefer gels and lotions over patches and injections.

As I mentioned earlier, the skin is water-proof, which means that gels and lotions will ‌sh off. Not only do topical solutions wash off, they rub off on clothing. You'll be getting less ‌your money if you use gels, lotions, creams or any other topical solution that aren't made ‌h liposome technology.

Gels and Lotions	
PROS	**CONS**
• Convenient • Inexpensive • Painless • Overusing is unlikely • Hormone levels are replenished at a pace your body can handle	• Can be a bit messy • You may experience an allergic reaction if you have exceptionally sensitive skin • Must be used daily

Remarkable Results

"My wife of 19 years regularly smothers her face with all ‌ds of creams, balsams, balms, conditioners and lotions. She said ‌helps reverse the aging process—utter decay. She's still lovely ‌thout these creams—a bit wrinkly, perhaps—but all these cold ‌eams in fancy jars are a marketing man's invention. None has ‌ne what they've promised except for the creams that are made ‌m liposomes. The effects are remarkable and I've monitored ‌r usage, only because I find the effects fascinating. I ask her if ‌e's been using the liposome cream. She's taken aback by the ‌ea that I've studied our bathroom cabinets so well."

—Eliyahu, 43

Benefits of "above-the-skin" bioidentical hormone delivery

Patches and Topical solutions: Gels, creams, lotions etc.

#1) Lowers the possibility of SHGB formation in the liver

#2) Bypasses the liver in the initial introduction of the natural supplemented hormones

#3) Ten times stronger than oral forms of delivery

#4) Can be customized specifically for your needs (i.e. dosage adjustment)

What is Liposome Technology?

Liposomes are able to cross the skin's barrier because it's the only form of gels or lotions that contain micro-encapsulation the skin can recognize. Liposomes are micro-encapsulated phosphatidylcholine. Skin and skin cells are also coated with phosphatidylcholine, which means your skin assumes that those liposomes are a part of its own.

Creams with liposomes are almost 1000 percent more effective than any other 24-hour time-released formula because bioidentical hormone gels and lotions are carried through the top layer of skin and transported into your blood. Additional studies have concluded that 95 percent of liposomes reach target cells by diffusing through the skin and entering through the blood stream.

In a 2002 study conducted at the University of Ljubljana, Slovenia, dermal therapy researchers concluded that liposomes "considerably improved the effectiveness of drugs," by "influencing the rate of transfer and efficacy of the drug's actions."

Pills, tablets and capsules

Despite a bad aftertaste, pills, tablets and capsules are effective. Oral consumption of any sort of bioidentical hormone supplement only requires a tall glass of water, making it a painless and a far quicker form of hormonal replacement delivery than injections or topical solutions.

Pills, tablets, and capsules	
PROS	**CONS**
• Convenient • Inexpensive • Painless • You can reduce or increase dosage depending on how you feel (i.e., if two pills a day aren't helping, you may want to try four; if four pills a day feels like it's too much, you can reduce it to three, and so on)	• Overdosing is a possibility • Oral consumption leads to minor SHGB formation (binding globulins resulting in less free anabolic hormones).

Sublingual Sprays	
PROS	**CONS**
• Bypasses the liver • Is transmitted directly into the blood • Convenient • Inexpensive • Painless • You can reduce or increase dosage depending on how you feel (i.e. if two sprays a day aren't helping, you may want to try four; if four sprays a day feels like it's too much, you can reduce it to three, and so on) • Is sprayed directly under the tongue; good for people who have trouble swallowing capsules • Suitable for traveling. You can take it with you everywhere, leave it in the office, keep it at home or stash in your purse.	• Overdosing is a possibility • Because the liver filters all oral supplements, you may exhaust it by taking pills, tablets or capsules for an extended period of time. • Oral consumption leads to the creation of SHGB.

Buyer Beware!

"Taking any estrogen orally even natural estrogen puts you at risk of accumulating too much estrogen in the liver. That stimulates the production of too many binding proteins (SHGB) which don't get just the estrogen, but, also, many other hormones making them inactive and creating other deficiencies," says Dr. Thierry Hertoghe in his book *The Hormone Solution: Stay younger longer with natural hormones and nutrition therapies* (Three Rivers Press, 2002).

Sublingual sprays

Last, but certainly not least, the sublingual spray is a popular method of hormone delivery for a variety of reasons. Just a few pumps under the tongue will give you your dosage for the day

What is First Pass Technology?

Like most cultural, personal and professional circles, medical crowds have their own jargon. Doctors refer to sublingual sprays and transdermal liposome creams as instruments of *First Pass Technology*. This means that transdermal liposome creams and to a lesser extent sublingual sprays, goes directly through the blood while bypassing the liver! That's right—no SHBGs with sublingual sprays! The natural bioidentical hormones go into the bloodstream through the vessels underneath your skin. This particular technology is shown to create less SHBG binding because the skin continuously absorbs much smaller amounts more closely to the physiological production of our own body.

✑ Dr. Tai's Secret ✑

To feel healthy and beautiful, you need to make sure your hormones are in balance. Each and every one of your symptoms will require a different dosage from a different hormone.

Emotional, physical and mental stressors can effect hormone consumption and absorption. If you've experienced a traumatic experience like a death in the family or job lay-off, you may require different dosages of a certain hormone. Contrary to this, if you've been in rather high spirits, you may require less of a dose. For example, if you've noticed the sex in your relationship has been getting better, you may be happier because you've become more active. In this case you may have to lower the dosage of hormonal supplementation only because your body has reached stabilization.

Please monitor your symptoms so you can adjust the dosage for your needs and your doctor can better understand what you need more or less of. But only you know your body the best and what you're feeling! So take personal responsibility and tell your doctor or health worker your symptoms and adjust your dosage accordingly.

CHAPTER 14

DHEA: Weapon against aging

Dean's War on Aging

"Losing my mind—literally, I was losing my mind! I began to forget things that were once so familiar to me. Birthdays used to be a cinch—I'd remember birthdays as I did faces. I realized something was wrong with me when I forgot the anniversary with my partner of four years. I thought maybe I was preoccupied, but I couldn't have been, because things really began to slow down at work. I run an online business and I'm always at home, so that wasn't the case. I've never been under insurmountable stress where it's affected my health or my state of mind. I've always been in control... until age hit me. Ironically, my doctor never made any mention that it could be my hormones until I saw a woman talk about her hormones on a daytime talk show. 'Alright,' I said to myself, 'I gotta check this out.'"

-Dean, 64

With more and more frequency, dehydroepiandrosterone (DHEA) is being added to the arsenal in the battle against aging. If you want to feel and look younger and better, consider taking a DHEA bioidentical supplement.

After several years on the market, DHEA is finally getting the recognition it deserves as it picks up momentum through marketing, advertising, and a surge of vitamins and supplements. Unlike other hormones such as HGH, DHEA is safe to use in physiologic does because the body has an abundance of it.

Where does it come from?

Like cortisol, the hormone DHEA is manufactured by the adrenal cortex, a small triangular gland that sits on top of both kidneys. After age 25, your body begins to lose approximately 2 percent of its DHEA every year. At age 50, your adrenals produce half the DHEA they once did. And by age 75, your DHEA levels are running on empty unless you do something to replenish them.

> ### Getting to know DHEA
>
> This anabolic hormone has actor-like characteristics. It's versatile and can take on a variety of roles at the same time by producing hormones while converting them into other hormones.
>
> Researchers have linked cancer to a lack of DHEA. Animal studies have shown that DHEA supplementation helped prevent obesity and memory loss and stimulate longevity.

Big Daddy

DHEA is considered the "father" among hormones just as the Pituitary gland is among glands. Together with pregnenolone (consider the mother of all hormones) affecting nearly every organ in our body including our brain, DHEA is an anabolic (protein building) hormone that possesses the ability to repair and construct tissues.

The multiple faces of DHEA

DHEA can be converted into testosterone, and oftentimes through aromatization it's converted into estradiol. DHEA and DHEA-S are mutually interchangeable through the process of sulfating; however, the concentration of DHEA is 500-1000 times lower than that of DHEA-S.

DHEA and its younger brother DHEA-S, which is a metabolized sulfate molecule from the liver, constantly work together in creating a balance for the body. Because DHEA can produce other hormones, supplemental DHEA takes on an especially important role in not just anti-aging medicine but in anti-obesity, anti-anxiety, anti-diabetes and a new one—anti-heart attacks.

What can DHEA do? (Ahlgrimm, M., The HRT Solution 1999; New York: Avery Pub.)

- Decreases blood cholesterol
- Decreases fatty deposit in blood vessel
- Lowers incidence of blood clots
- Improves bone growth
- Supports weight loss
- Improves brain function
- Improves sense of well being
- Supports your immune system
- Improves cell repair
- Decreases allergic reactions
- Allows better stress management

> **DHEA shows hope**
>
> Studies conducted on rabbits at Johns Hopkins University in 1988 have shown that supplemental DHEA improved the severity of arteriosclerosis. Results showed nearly 50 percent of plaque shrinkage in the inner lining of blood vessels. These very same clinical studies have shown that higher levels of DHEA confer improvement in cardiovascular protection for men as they did in rabbits.

Breast Cancer

Dr. Bulbrook from
England reported
that women
developing breas
cancer have very
low levels of DHEA
These low levels o
DHEA can appear
much as nine year
prior to the diagnos
of breast cancer. D
Bulbrook found in a
study of 5000 wome
that 27 women
developed breast
cancer because
they had low level:
of DHEA.

DHEA and the aging man

During andropause, DHEA serves as a powerful androgen formation, supportive of producing natural testosterone in the body. It can have a positive effect on aging men suffering from:

- declining muscle mass
- increased body fat around the waist and the middle of the body
- libido reduction
- fatigue
- dry skin
- energy loss
- strength loss

The possibility of bringing health and happiness to all aging males significantly increases by using DHEA replacement with its positive effect on testosterone production. By supplementing with bioidentical DHEA, men will turn into lovers instead of fighters.

DHEA and the aging woman

Women will greatly benefit from DHEA replacement because of its powerful anti-depressant and anti-anxiety effects. If you're a woman and you're reading this, I know you'll find it especially interesting that DHEA will improve libido and boost your skin's thickness and collagen.

Supplemental DHEA optimizes improvement in serum estrogen as well as testosterone in women, according to a study conducted in 2000 by Dr. Baulieu. Estrogen, a major female sex hormone, plays a big part in how sexually active a woman is and how firm her skin is.

After testing DHEA's effects on a group of women, Dr. Baulieu found that they reported having a greater desire to have sex more often, which was probably due to the development of more energy, therefore greater self-esteem (energy and self-esteem go hand-in-hand (Baulieu, E.E., et al. "DHEA Sulfate and aging contribution of the DHEA age study to socio-biomedical." *Proceedings from the National Academy of Sciences USA*, 2000; 97(8)4279-4284).

DHEA Benefits (*Lieberman, S., The Real Vitamin and Mineral Book. NY: Avery Pub. 1997*)

Increases muscle strength and lean body mass

2.   Improves immune function

3.   Improves quality of life

4.   Improves sleep

5.   Boosts feelings of wellness

6.   Decreases joint pain

7.   Improves sensitivity to insulin

8.   Lowers fatty triglycerides

9.   Prevents damaging effects of stress

Can DHEA protect against cancer?

Case study #1

A number of reports suggest that DHEA has an extraordinarily positive effect on cancer. By gathering cell cultures, Dr. Arthur Schwartz of Temple University saw the amazing results DHEA had on cancer patients. He noted that when cancer patients were given DHEA through their diet, the cells which were unaffected by cancer became stronger.

> **DHEA Bonus**
>
> Research conducted at the University of California, San Diego among 1029 patients showed a significant reduction (up to 25 percent) in the risk of cardiovascular disease in men.

Inspired by this, Dr. Schwartz conducted further research using mice that were predisposed to breast cancer. He found that the mice without DHEA suffered and most of them died, while the mice that had been supplemented with DHEA were free of tumors.

Dr. Schwartz conducted two additional studies in 1981 and 1984 on two separate and different strains of mice where he found a 75 percent and 100 percent reduction in cancer after 8 months. In one of the studies which spanned 15 months, he found a 50-75 percent reduction in the cancer rate among these mice.

Dr. Schwartz concluded that DHEA supplementation protected mice from forming cancer in tissues, skin, lungs, breasts, intestines and the liver. (Schwartz, Arthur. "Cancer prevention with DHEA." *Journal of Cellular Biochemistry*, 1995; 59(S22):210-217.)

Case study #2

In 1999, Dr. McCormich and Dr. Rao found that rats supplemented with DHEA and exposed to cancer seemed to be resistant to further developing other forms of cancer (e.g. prostate cancer).

The doctors stated in their study that "DHEA inhibits prostate cancer induction both when chronic administration is begun prior to carcinogen exposure, and when administration is delayed until pre-neoplastic prostate lesions are present."

DHEA works as an effective contributor to prostate cancer prevention, concluded the two authors. (McCormick, D. L. and Rao, K.V.N., et al. "Chemoprevention of hormone dependent prostate cancer in wistar unilever rats." *The Journal of European Urology*, 1999; 35: 464-467.)

So how can DHEA bioidentical supplementation help you?

1) It can have a protective effect against accumulation of visceral fat and development of muscle. DHEA also shows insulin resistance in rats fed a high-fat diet.

(*American Journal of Physiology*, November, 1997; 273(5 pt 2): R1704-8.)

2) In DHEA studies, serum levels were restored to those found in young adults (25+) within two weeks of DHEA replacement.

In women, DHEA increased serum levels of androgens (androstenedione, testosterone and dehydrotestosterone).

In men, there was a small rise of androstenedione. Perceived physical and psychological well-being rose by 67 percent in men and 84 percent in women.

(*Journal of Clinical Endocrinology and Metabolism*, June 1994; 78(6): 1360)

3) DHEA is a steroid that blocks carcinogenensis, retards aging, and exerts antiproliferative aging properties. Low levels of DHEA are linked to an increase of developing cancer or cardiovascular disease. High levels of DHEA inhibit the development of atherosclerosis.

(*Journal of Clinical Investigations*, **August, 1998; 82(2): 712-20**)

ral vs. Transdermal Delivery: Which method is best for DHEA pplementation?

Ils and Tablets

DHEA tablets are inexpensive and are commonly
ailable throughout pharmacies, grocery stores and local
alth food stores. However, some research indicates that
al consumption of DHEA may lead to the following
mplications:

> **Protect Your Heart**
>
> • DHEA can significantly minimize progression of cardiovascular disease on an older aging population.
>
> • High levels of DHEA may retard the development of coronary atherosclerosis and coronary vasculopathy. (*Annals of New York Academy of Sciences*, December, 1995; 774:271-80.)

1) DHEA causes the liver a great deal of stress because it isn't easily digested. Taken orally, DHEA travels through the stomach, into mesenteric arteries, and finally to the liver where it's metabolized. Between 90 and 95 percent of DHEA will be filtered and discarded by the liver, leaving you with no more that 5 to 10 percent of usable DHEA.

2) Through oral consumption of DHEA, sex hormone binding globulins becomes a greater threat and complication. When taken orally in large doses, DHEA causes an alarm to go off in the liver, whereupon the sex hormone binding globulin* (SHBG) may go into hyper production, tripling the level in order for the liver to neutralize excess DHEA.

Naturally, the liver doesn't know any better. All it knows is that it is being bombarded and overwhelmed by DHEA so it will do what it does best, which is neutralizing excessive hormonal amounts.

he problem with SHBG outpour is that SHBG doesn't really know or care what hormone is being ided, so it may end up binding not just DHEA but also testosterone and other essential hormones.

Technology to the rescue!

Clearly, the best approach for DHEA supplementation is via First Pass Technology-- or transdermal liposomes. Through this mechanism, DHEA is protected by micro encapsulation of liposome and instantaneously absorbed and delivered through the sub-dermal vasculature. Tablets and pills take several hours to be metabolized by the liver, whereas with liposomes, DHEA is transported directly into the bloodstream where it can be disposed of within minutes.

Research proves that........... *DHEA should be transdermal.*

Because....

In an experiment performed by Dr. C. Labrie (et al.), she concluded that the transdermal route of delivery was ten times more effective than the oral route. Dr. Labrie and her researchers stated that her data shows high bioavailability of percutaneous DHEA as measured by its androgenic biological activities. (Labrie, C. and Belanger, A., et al. "High bioavailability of DHEA administered percutaneously in the rat." *Journal of Endocrinology*, 1996; 150: S107-118.)

In addition, a variety of other studies show that transdermal administration of DHEA on postmenopausal women for six months resulted in significantly increased density and mineralization of the hip bone. This has a positive effect on osteoblastic activity of bone, and has clinical uses such as increasing supplementation of DHEA for osteoporosis. Some authors have reported that an increase in DHEA levels will lower the rate of accidents caused by osteoporosis.

DHEA Checklist	
You may have a DHEA deficiency if you answer yes to any of these questions:	**You may have an excess of DHEA if you answer yes to any of these questions:**
❑ Do you feel depressed? ❑ Are you having problems handling stress? ❑ Do you have a lack of stamina? ❑ Are you moody? ❑ Do you have dry eyes? ❑ Do you have osteoporosis? ❑ Are you experiencing memory loss? ❑ Do you have bone, muscle, or joint pain?	❑ Are you growing facial hair? ❑ Is your skin oily? ❑ Do you have acne pimples? ❑ Are you being bossy? ❑ Are you impatient/anger? ❑ Are you easily irritated? ❑ Is your voice deepening?
If supplementation has already been taken, *increase* your dosage if you experience the above symptoms.	If supplementation has already been taken, *decrease* your dosage if you experience the above symptoms.

How much DHEA should you take?

DHEA is produced by the adrenal gland and is at its highest level early in the morning. The best physiological approach for DHEA supplementation is to apply transdermal DHEA early in the morning, upon waking.

Daily supplementation of DHEA is a vital and powerful program for anti-aging hormonal balance. It stimulates the androgenic repair function of DHEA hormone. You can start with 25 to 50 mg of transdermal DHEA daily, and adjust the dosage as needed.

Your goal should be to maintain a physiologic DHEA level equivalent to that of a 30 to 35-year-old person. Customize the dosage to how much you require, but most importantly, how much you can tolerate.

Again, I'd like to remind you that an excess of DHEA (or any other hormone) can be potentially dangerous. Every few months, your family physician or health care worker should make sure that you're taking appropriate levels of bioidentical supplementation by testing your DHEA levels.

ꙮ Dr. Tai's Secret ꙮ

One of the best-kept secrets in your fight against aging is DHEA supplementation. Not only does DHEA serve as a protector for your brain, immune and cardiovascular systems, bioidentical supplementation of the hormone helps to make us happy by keeping our energy levels high.

Bioidentical supplementation will also improve your well-being and give you a greater ability to cope with chronic stress that could potentially accelerate aging. DHEA has been researched and clearly shown to work well with cortisol (stress hormone; preventing adrenal fatigue). DHEA is certainly one of the most powerful protective and anti-aging hormones we have at our disposal. Make sure your DHEA levels are equivalent to biologically aged 35-year-old's. If it is, you can kiss your lack of energy, libido loss and stress good-bye!

CHAPTER 15

Pregnenolone

"I've always asked myself, what good am I if I can no longer make contributions to the world? What good am I if I can no longer teach or learn or give? Who am I if I can't remember my family, my past, and my experiences?"

--Dr. Tai

W ithout a functioning mind, we are, in a sense, useless.

As everyday passes, we all age--nobody gets any younger. And despite the fact that at times I wish I could freeze time for myself, I wouldn't wish to stop the hands of time for anyone else. I want my grandchild to grow; I want to see her become a high school graduate, a college graduate, a mother, a beautiful woman. I want to see my students become successful doctors; I want to hear about the lives they've saved. I want to live long enough to see everyone's successes and experience their stories as they're told. I want to experience all of these things so badly that I've realized that getting old isn't so bad, just as long as I can remember everything.

No cholesterol....no hormone production

If hormones evolved like life evolved on earth, pregnenolone would be a dinosaur. It's one of the oldest hormones and has had the longest lifespan within a person's body. Directly derived from cholesterol, pregnenolone helps convert over 150 steroid hormones. For this reason, people that want to lower their cholesterol levels should proceed with caution because without cholesterol, there would virtually be no hormone production.

People with low cholesterol levels generally have a pregnenolone deficiency, and they are likely to suffer from symptoms that affect the preservation of memories and illnesses of the brain such as Alzheimer's, dementia and senility.

If hormones had a family hierarchy, cholesterol would be Grandmother (Source) and pregnenolone would be Mother, the one that all the other hormone family members come from

Where does pregnenolone come from?

When cholesterol is synthesized from the liver and changed in the adrenal cortex (the two glands that sit above the kidneys), it creates pregnenolone. As with all of your other hormones, pregnenolone production slows with age. When pregnenolone levels drop, the outlook is grim, because pregnenolone provides the materials for other hormones to grow and multiply in number.

> **Something to think about**
>
> The word "pregnenolone" has the prefix of "preg-" like pregnant. It births other hormones like a woman does a child.

Pregnenolone—a stress reliever?

Pregnenolone, like cortisol (also produced in the adrenal glands), works diligently to improve our body's ability to deal with stress. As you probably already know, stress is extremely destructive because of its potential to cause a compilation of diseases and symptoms that can shorten our lives and destroy our health.

Curious as to how pregnenolone produces calming effects, Dr. Hans Selye, a pioneer in research, conducted studies in 1943 on mice and then on humans. Dr. Selye wrote in a study published in the *Pineal Journal Review*, "Pregnenolone hormone reduces stress and fatigue by repairing the damages of stress and fatigue."

What Dr. Selye meant by that was stress, like a torn shirt, tears easily once someone has initiated a rip. If you've already experienced stress to the greatest extent, it's most likely had a negative effect on your body which you were unable to mend. By adding more stress, you're worsening the damage. By using a supplement that lowers stress, you're repairing damages while preventing potentially volatile future reactions.

Dr. Selye explained that pregnenolone was able to control the damaging effects of stress through neutralizing excess cortisol. The overproduction of cortisol, he said, is the result of relentless stress and abnormalities in metabolizing sugar. Thus, replenishing depleted pregnenolone can help you avoid severe depression and all of the other symptoms associated with too much cortisol such as water retention, insomnia, over-eating, weakened immunities and destabilized liver functions. (Selye, H., et al. "Potentiation of a pituitary extract with pregnenolone and additional observations concerning the influence of various organs on steroids, metabolism." *Pineal Journal Review*, 1943; 10(2):319-28.)

Memory like an elephant or......a mouse?

Besides helping people cope with stress, pregnenolone affects the brain more than anything. Decades ago, in the 1940s, researchers obsessed over pregnenolone (they had every right to). Their curiosity of the parent hormone led them to discovering something miraculous in a laboratory filled with white little mice.

One group of mice was left alone, while the others were injected with pregnenolone. The group injected with pregnenolone made their way through a maze faster than the group that wasn't injected. Do you want to know why the injected mice got to the finish line before the mice that were left alone? Sure you do. After conducting a few of the same studies, the researchers concluded that pregnenolone helped the mice remember their way around the maze! This led the researchers to believe that pregnenolone has a lot to do with the brain's most sophisticated roles — memory.

Recently, because of data that's been collected over decades of research, pregnenolone has been proven to contribute to increased intelligence, learning, memory and alertness.

> **Good to Know**
>
> A diet consisting of too much saturated fat and trans-fatty acids interferes and blocks with the natural pathway of pregnenolone. (*Yanick, P., Prohormone Nutrition, Montclair, NJ:Longevity Institute International, 1998.*)

Pregnenolone Benefits

1.   Improves excitation and inhibition of the nervous system.

2.   Increases resistance to stress

3.   Improves physical and mental energy

4.   Increases nerve transmission and memory

5.   Reduces pain and inflammation

:

Clear as day

By having higher levels of pregnenolone, you're able to think clearer by recalling information with less delay. This was shown in 1992 when researcher J.F. Flood (et al.) tested the memory enhancing effects in male mice using pregnenolone and steroids metabolically derived from it. He found that pregnenolone helps the neurotransmission of the nerves speak to each other. When reviewed, his study read that neurons communicate with each other through electrochemical. (Flood, J. F., et al. "Memory-enhancing effects in male mice of pregnenolone and steroids metabolically derived from it." *Proceedings from the National Academy of Science of the United State of America*, 1992; 89:1567-71).

Pregnenolone and mental illness

Not only does bioidentical pregnenolone supplementation play an important role in preserving one's memory, it has also been shown to be effective against depression. McGavack, a researcher in the early '50s, found that pregnenolone was lower in individuals who were diagnosed with mental and emotional disorders.

McGavack helped patients undergoing internal kismet by placing them on a bioidentical pregnenolone supplementation plan. Weeks after supplementation, McGavack found that his patients weren't as depressed. (McGavack, T., et al. "The use of pregnenolone in various clinical disorders." *Journal of Clinical Endocrinology and Metabolism*, 1951; 11: 559-77.)

Guess what else pregnenolone can do?

- In addition to controlling stress, pregnenolone has been studied on its positive effects directly correlated to arthritis. Pregnenolone has been found to help with swelling, inflammation, joint and muscle pain—most, if not all, of the symptoms related to arthritis. (Freeman, H., et al. "Therapeutic efficacy of pregnenolone in rheumatoid arthritis." *The Journal of the American Medical Association*, 1950; 143: 338-44.)

- In addition to helping patients control arthritis, researcher R. Davison (et al.) found that pregnenolone supplementation has had helpful effects on immune diseases lupus and psoriasis. (Davison, R., et al. "Effects of pregnenolone on rheumatoid arthritis." *Archives of Internal Medicine*, 1950; 85: 365-88.)

Pregnenolone Checklist	
You may have a pregnenolone deficiency if you answer yes to any of these questions:	**You may have an excess of pregnenolone if you answer yes to any of these questions:**
❑ Do you feel depressed? ❑ Do you have short-term memory loss? ❑ Are you forgetful? ❑ Is your thinking kind of fuzzy? ❑ Are colors not so bright? ❑ Are you more pessimistic?	❑ Are you feeling edgy? ❑ Are you feeling uptight? ❑ Do you frequently worry?
If supplementation has already been taken, *increase* your dosage if you experience the above symptoms.	If supplementation has already been taken, *decrease* your dosage if you experience the above symptoms.

Pregnenolone Supplementation

Combining DHEA and pregnenolone together seems to be a lot more effective than just using pregnenolone alone. Together, I've found that DHEA and pregnenolone are profoundly well received by the adrenal cortex as well as the rest of the body. Pregnenolone and DHEA should be used in the form of a liposome cream. This way, the application is absorbed transdermally, so it avoids your liver, therefore, causing no rebound effects and a reduced likelihood of over-consuming, so you don't experience the side effects previously mentioned (tension, edginess, and anxiousness).

🐉 Dr. Tai's Secret 🐉
It's important to remember that the body is made up of both male and female hormones. Pregnenolone is the base of all of these hormones—therefore, it is crucial (regardless of your sex) that everyone replenishes lost pregnenolone levels. Because of age, some people may require more than others, but nevertheless, pregnenolone is the first hormone that you should be concerned with, and it's the first hormone that you should seek to replenish. For a sharp memory, decreased mental fatigue, better stress adaptation, and enhanced concentration, I suggest you try adding pregnenolone to your bioidentical hormone replacement program to sharpen your memory and improve your vitality.

CHAPTER 16

HGH – The Fountain of Youth

"Health is a state of complete harmony of the body, mind and spirit. "

~B.K.S. Iyengar

When Ponce de Leon set off to sail the seven seas in search of the awe-inspiring Fountain of Youth, he inevitably failed, instead discovering one of our 50 states (not so bad for failure). Hundreds of years have passed since his quest, and for just as long, we, as people, have mimicked the Spanish explorer by conducting our own personal quests of striving to find ways to *Feel Stronger, Look Younger and Live Longer.*

The Fountain of Youth does exist. It may not be a body of water in a wild rainforest or a magical potion, but it does indeed exist. This legendary youth-restoring antidote is nothing more than a hormone replacement system with its most powerful hormone being HGH, the human growth hormone.

When HGH fizzles out

After childhood, HGH levels peak and then your body will maintain a low level of HGH throughout the rest of your life. Without this hormone, age begins to look like it sucks out every ounce of resilience from us. Like blood in a glass of water, it curls and works its way throughout the interior of the glass turning the water pink. Age does something similar, and it affects every part and portion of our bodies. Contrary to cliché, age discriminates as it seems to concentrate on our face. Nevertheless, it also takes a toll on our body by shrinking muscles, bones and blood vessels, causing us to make conscious effort to do the simplest of things like standing up straight. Anti-aging involves more than just your exterior—it requires reshaping your interior.

How is HGH made?

HGH is made in the pituitary gland, deep inside the brain just behind the eyes. It's a microscopic protein substance that is secreted in short pulses during the first hours of sleep and after exercise. Produced throughout a person's lifetime, there is no shortage of HGH during youth. It stimulates growth in children and plays an important role in adult metabolism.

It's a simple protein made of 191 chain amino acids that are in a polypeptide formation. HGH is responsible for controlling most of the major functions in our bodies. It's especially important to know that as a peptide, its delicate nature is overly sensitive and can be destroyed by gastric acid found in saliva and stomach acids.

Chante's Story

"I've used human growth hormone for a year and six months. Since I've used HGH, I've lost weight and am convinced it helped my skin. It's done something to me and my nieces tell me every day. I've had the energy to do what I want; I don't make any more excuses and have seen that I've been more outgoing.

Although I love kids, I was unhappy working at the same high school as a secretary. Eight years ago, after my partner died, r love for dogs grew exceedingly. My two retrievers have given me the company and love I need. A little while after notifying the scho of my leave, I decided to take up dog training courses.

I'm now two months away from be a certified dog trainer I'm very excited, and have, in a way, started over again. I feel like a new woman and that's a good feeling. If it wasn't for the HGH and various other bioidentical hormones, at age 64, I don't think I wou have developed the courage or confidence to do what I did. Instea of retiring, I went to school and started a career I know I'll excel i

Manufactured in the anterior frontal lobe of the pituitary gland (a small pea-sized gland located at the base of the brain), HGH is secreted in large waves and spurts around the time you fall asleep. HGH's most intense activity occurs between 10 p.m. and 4 a.m. Its production is closely related and affected by the Human growth release Hormone (HGRH).

Benefits of HGH

Adults who take human growth factors have said that they feel younger, more sociable and have a greater desire to be active. Literally, HGH impacts every cell in our body as a "master hormone"; it's what makes us grow. Other benefits include:

- Increased energy
- Amplified muscle mass
- Greater cardiac input
- Enhanced memory

- Enhanced libido
- Increased fat burning
- Stronger bones and muscles
- Enhanced immune system
- Increased agility

- Better sleep
- Improved cholesterol profile
- Sharper vision
- Hair regrowth
- Thicker skin

- Lower blood pressure
- Improved social skills

- Rapid wound healing
- Increased sense of well-being

More good news

According to a 1999 study published in the New England Journal of Medicine, after six months of treatment, metabolism increased by 6 percent to 11 percent. In addition, it was found that HGH restores normal body composition, improves muscle tone and normalizes serum lipid concentrations. Overall, HGH improves quality of life, including: energy level, mood and emotions. (*New England Journal of Medicine*, October 1999; 341:1206-1216.)

Meet the Growth Hormones

When HGH is released, it moves through the bloodstream and is taken to tissues, where specific receptor sites in organs throughout the body are identified and then locked in. There's a specific key-and-lock relationship where growth hormones are attracted to certain receptor sites. Most of human growth hormones are delivered into the liver where the liver cells (through its metabolic process) convert it into insulin growth factor-1 (IGF-1) and five other growth hormones: epidermal growth factor (EGF), vascular growth factor (VGF), nerve growth factor (NGF), transfer growth factor (TGF) and insulin growth factor 2 (IGF-2).

When IGF-1 levels fall below the adult normal range of 200 to 500 ng/ml, muscle and bone strength and energy levels most likely will decrease. Tissue repair, cell re-growth, healing capacity, upkeep of vital organs, brain and memory function, enzyme production, and revitalization of hair, nails and skin will also diminish. While aging and decreasing growth hormone levels go hand-in-hand, those who lose their pituitary production of HGH due to surgery, infection or an accident, instantly suffer many profound ill effects.

Did you know?

HGH decreases by 75 percent from adulthood to midlife. HGH loss is complete by age 40. (*The Journal of the American Medical Association*, August, 2000; 284(7): 861-866.)

Growth hormone has important effects on protein, lipid and carbohydrate metabolism. By age 50, half of the growth factors levels are depleted; by 80, almost everything is gone.

Turning back the hands of time

HGH is an important tool to adding years to your life along with rejuvenating your body physically and mentally. With less than a year of treatment, studies have shown that medically supervised HGH therapies can turn back the clock on the effects of aging by as much as 10 to 20 years.

HGH and Obesity

Low dose growth hormone treatment with diet restriction accelerates body fat loss, exerts anabolic effect and improves growth hormone secretory dysfunction in obese adults. *Kim KR, et al. Horm Res 1999; 511(2) :78-8.*

HGH deficiency

Some researchers believe that an HGH deficiency causes lower self-esteem, which may lead to depression and social isolation. Pessimistic perceptions on the self can negatively impact relationships both in the home and office, e.g. quitting a job or breaking up with partners, friends and spouses.

An HGH deficiency results in lower bone mineral density, lower bone mineral content and therefore increased risk of osteoporosis and osteomalacia.

Growth hormone production drops at least 15 percent every ten years. As you lose HGH, you lose an equal amount of IGF-1. Once you lose HGH and IGF-1, concentrating becomes difficult and you'll most definitely lose the desire for more physical activities like having sex and exercising. You'll begin to see a different you-- a lazier, fatter, more depressed version of   yourself.

HGH Instant Replay

- The liver converts HGH into an insulin factor also known as somatomedin-C into six additional growth factors: IGF-1, IGF-2, EGF, NGF, TGF and VGF.
- Children have approximately more or less of 600 ml, while adults have less than 200 ml of HGH.
- If IGF-1 falls, muscle and bone mass fall.

Because of decreased cardiac output, heart X-rays show that an HGH-deficient patient has reduced left ventricle mass and a decreased shortening of the heart muscle. The exercise capacity in a person lacking HGH (which probably includes all of us) is 25 percent less than those who have abundant amounts of HGH hence muscle mass and muscle strength loss is also predominant.

HGH pills, shots or what??

It doesn't matter how clever an advertisement is – don't fall for HGH in a pill, because it doesn't come in a pill! Most often, HGH is injected. Human growth hormone can only be obtained through prescription injections from your physician. After you've consulted your physician, he or she will give you a prescription for an HGH injectable divided into dosages per week. Smaller amounts are considered to be safer. You may inject HGH using hypodermic diabetic syringes along the sides of your stomach (sides nearest to your bellybutton).

While pinching your skin, you can inject yourself every night when you go to bed or early in the morning when you wake up. Some doctors will recommend 2 or 3 shots throughout the day. This is entirely up to you, give it a shot (ha-ha!) and check it out!

Your doctor will give you guidelines, but only you can evaluate the side effects. Be sure to give your doctor feedback. With this information, both you and your doctor will be able to decide if you should increase or decrease the units injected. After letting ample time pass since administering your injections, make sure you have your physician monitor your IGH-1 and IGF binding globulin 3 (IGFBP-3).

HGH turns muscle into fat

In a study conducted with 24 HGH-deficient adults over a six-month period, there was marked improvement in lean body mass when a minimal amount of HGH was administered. Researchers concluded that HGH increased positive protein synthesis, thus improving muscle mass and muscle function as well as muscle strength. In these patients, there was a significant decline in fat mass around soft internal organs (visceral) as well as around the waist, compared to the arms, neck and legs. Without exercise, patients lost over 3 kilos (6 pounds) of fat within that period and gained 3 kilos of muscle!

Injections aren't just painful

Due to the normal physiology of the human body to produce frequent hourly small spurts of human growth hormone to be converted into IGF-1, once-daily injections do not emulate nature and therefore tend to produce serious side effects such as carpal tunnel syndrome, arthritis, joint pain, water retention and hypertension.

Many doctors are trying to lower the dosages of human growth hormone per day to get the maximum benefit with the least amount of side effects. Reports of therapeutic benefits are mixed, with some people experiencing fabulous results, while others who were looking for weight loss did not get what they expected for the trouble and cost.

Growth hormone is a very powerful hormone which can have bad side effects if taken incorrectly. It is not, however, a dangerous hormone if it is taken correctly and the results are closely monitored. Incorrect usage could result in harmful side effects such as: water retention, prostate pain and carpal tunnel syndrome.

Edema

Retention of water or edema isn't as serious a side effect as one would expect. Edema disappears if dosage is lowered or after the body adjusts to the increase in growth hormone.

Carpal tunnel syndrome

Carpal tunnel syndrome is a painful condition in the wrist caused by small bones rubbing against each other. It occurs after a few months of taking too much growth hormone. This symptom is preventable by monitoring the results of taking growth hormone, and is normally reversible by discontinuing or lowering the dose being taken.

Gigantism

A tremendous excess in growth hormone could lead to a horrible disease known as acromegaly, or gigantism, which is an unnatural growth of bone mass and thickening of the skin. In persons that have a pituitary tumor, acromegaly occurs naturally because growth hormones are released without control.

Human Growth Matrix—an HGH alternative

Although it isn't HGH in the purest form, Human Growth Matrix is pretty darn close. It's a sublingual spray with all the growth factors you'll need and you can take this supplement in the morning and at night. Spritz—once in the a.m. and twice in the p.m.

What is Human Growth Matrix made of?

Considered to be a technology breakthrough, Human Growth Matrix is formulated from natural water extracted from deer antler, which is a natural source of IGF-1 that is known to keep people young. Emperors and members of the nobility have been using deer antler for ages. In the last 25 years, much effort has been put forth by a number of scholarly institutions to research and extract IGF-1 from deer antler. Through special water extraction, IGF-1 has been extracted from deer antler successfully.

How does Human Growth Matrix work?

Human Growth Matrix (see sources) is a microencapsulation of natural IGF-1 from a water extraction of deer antler in a liposome carrier that is sprayed sublingually. By spraying under the tongue, your blood absorbs it in the upper GI tract where it doesn't get digested and broken by the digestive acids and juices.

Human Growth Matrix is a new and improved delivery system of liposomes. Using nanotechnology, delivering HGH has never been so available or affordable. You get the benefits of human growth factor without the expense or the inconvenience of HGH injections.

For specific conditions like severe arthritis, traumatic injury or inflammation, you may want to increase the human growth matrix dosage to three or four spray pumps, once in the morning and twice in the evening to help with inflammation and pain control.

Be smart!

Not only is it necessary to take blood tests to monitor results, it is also foolish to take a dose much above what is the normal physiological standard. At the start of a program, taking 1 i.u. per day of HGH is the most you should take unless your doctor advises more, and you should not increase this dose unless you take a saliva test that shows you can safely increase your dose.

HGH Checklist	
You may have a HGH deficiency if you answer yes to any of these questions:	**You may have an excess of HGH if you answer yes to any of these questions:**
❑ Are you gaining fat around your waist and hips? ❑ Are you losing muscle? ❑ Is your strength decreasing? ❑ Are you more tired? ❑ Do you have bone and joint pain? ❑ Have you lost interest in sex? ❑ Have you become anti-social? ❑ Is your skin thin, saggy, and wrinkly? ❑ Has your libido decreased?	❑ Are you suffering from carpal tunnel syndrome? ❑ Do you have sudden arthritis pain? ❑ Are you retaining water? ❑ Do you have high blood pressure? ❑ Do you have prostate pain or is it enlarged? ❑ Are you exhibiting aggressive behavior?
If supplementation has already been taken, *increase* your dosage if you experience the above symptoms.	If supplementation has already been taken, *decrease* your dosage if you experience the above symptoms.

♌ Dr. Tai's Secret ♎

It's well known that as we age there is also a decrease of HGH affecting all the hormones functions on the body, organ, and metabolism. Overall, these have general magnifying effects on our bodies. As we age, we lose tissue hydration and water from our body. Therefore, we actually see visible signs of winkles and dry skin. If you compare a young person's body water content with that of an elderly person, you will notice over 10 to 14 percent less water content in the tissues, skin and body of the elderly. This is a huge difference with extraordinary consequences. With HGH replacement, one of the beneficial effects is the potential improvement in skin, tissues, organ and joint hydration. HGH replacement can cause your skin to become so plump and moist you won't be able to keep yourself from reminiscing about "the good old days."

However, if you overdose on HGH, you could develop hypertension, joint pain, water retention and swelling, and those are just some of the less serious cases. HGH is not hormone you want to mess around with. Therefore, use a minimum amount for tissue water content and optimum hydration.

Finally, if you suffer from cancer, are in remission, or have a family history of cancer, HGH and IGF-1 is not for you! We don't have clinical evidence of any conflict between HGH/IGF-1 and cancer therapies; in fact, we have just the opposite. Multiple studies show no cancerous effects from IGF-1. Nevertheless, as a precaution, I suggest not to use either HGH or IGF-1 if you have a history of cancer

CHAPTER 17

Testosterone

"Make the most of yourself, for that is all there is of you."

~Ralph Waldo Emerson

Testosterone has long been recognized as the hormone of desire; it helps to transform boys into sexually functional men. But testosterone isn't just for men, it's also very important to a woman as well. In fact, without testosterone, there would be no "woman." Our bodies essentially depend on the production of an adequate level of testosterone to create all the positive traits that we need as men and as women. Testosterone production is the end result of a long chain of events that starts way up in the center of our brain.

Roman's story

"For some reason, I had always thought that it was OK to be overweight if no one was going to see you naked. It has been at least five years since I've been to the beach and my wife and I haven't been intimate in months.

For a while, my wife Ava and I were going through some pretty rough times. In fact, we used to sleep in separate bedrooms. I used to think we stayed together for the same reasons most people stay together—the kids and out of convenience. We really don't understand each other, but we do know and respect each other. I'm loyal because I have no desire to be intimate with anyone. I think if I was physically capable to show someone I love them, I'd try to make love to my wife.

Unlike many of my friends who've tried erection formulas, I was just too embarrassed to give them a shot, especially since I've heard claims about heart failure in men. I tried putting myself on a strict diet by excluding sugars from snacks and meals, and then I finally went to my doctor when I wasn't getting anywhere. My doctor informed me that my testosterone level was

---

A piece of history

In 1889, Charles Edouard Brown-Sequard, a French physiologist, injected an extract made from guinea pig and dog testicles into himself. Sequard wasn't aware of what he was injecting until he felt the combination's after-effects. Days later, he felt sharper and stronger. In his memoirs, he noted that he had increased mental energy by recalling things he thought he'd forgotten. Soon enough, Sequard realized that he felt the way he did because of the chemicals within the animal's gonads. Needless to say, since then, testosterone has become a well-known hormone.

down. All it took was a glance at my chest size and my large, wide waist and hips. I asked him if there was anything that could be done and he said that he could offer me synthetic testosterone or natural testosterone. Wanting to know which was best, I asked for a list of pros and cons, and from what I gathered, it seemed as if he preferred natural testosterone.

I decided to use the natural testosterone and I've lost inches all over my body, plus I'm still continuing to lose. I'm 5-foot-11-inches tall and used to weigh 258—today I weigh 206. I've lost my breasts and I feel more energetic. I feel like I'm in my 20s all over again. I can't wait to see how I evolve months from now and I can't wait to find out what the new me does to our relationship."

--Roman, 45

What goes up, comes down

While testosterone isn't the only male hormone (androgen), it is the predominant ruler within a man's body. This is why men tend to have a larger build, larger bone structures, broader shoulders and more facial hair than women.

For men, the Leydig cells in the testes produce about 3 to 10 mg of testosterone each day. During puberty, testosterone peaks, and then these levels start declining after age 25. Every ten years after 25, you can count on losing more than 10 percent of your testosterone levels, and by 80, you'll have less than 10 percent of what you once had. The most abrupt changes in testosterone levels start around age 40. Like a roller-coaster, you ride all way up to the top — this is testosterone production during adolescence. Then while still securely fastened into your seat, you feel the descent. After 40, you start to pick up momentum, basically freefalling down to the bottom, and by 80, you're back to where you started — the same amount you had when you were a child.

In women, testosterone is secreted by the ovaries and adrenals. Throughout a female's puberty, she produces increased amounts of testosterone, which is the precursor to estrogen. A woman's testosterone levels are highest in her early twenties and begin to decline when estrogen levels start dropping during the first stages of menopause.

Physicians tend to see most effects of testosterone deficiency as a woman approaches and enters menopause. Because the ovaries produce the majority of testosterone and estrogens, testosterone, estrone, and estradiol levels will be lower if a woman has her ovaries removed either for medical or personal reasons.

With the cessation of 80% of hormonal production, a peri- menopausal woman suffers from estrogen, progesterone and testosterone deficiency.

What does testosterone do anyway?

1) Increases your sexual desire and libido

2) Stimulates feelings of emotional well-being, self-

confidence, and motivation. Persky, H., Arch Sex Behav 1978; 7(3): 157-173

3) Increases muscle mass and strength

4) Responsible for growth of pubic and underarm hair

5) Improves memory. Vliet, E. Women, Weight and Hormones, NY;

M. Evans & Company 2001

6) Improves muscle tone and sagging skin. Brincat, M.,Br. Med. J. 1983; 287(6402): 1337-1338

7) Decreases body fat

8) Prevents osteoporosis. Davis, S., Curr Opin Obstet Gynecol 1997; 9(3); 177-180

Andropause, such a cruel reality!!!

Testimonial

"I lost a lot of the hair on my head, and I started losing the hair on my arms, underneath my arms, all over my body and even my eyebrow hair started to thin. It was a very sad time in my life, because beside the curves on a woman's body, I feel that a woman's hair defines her. Because I barely had any left, I couldn't do anything with my hair. I was relieved to find that I wasn't diseased—instead I had extremely low testosterone and thyroid."-

Barbara, 56

In the U.S., 5 million men suffer from the "cruel reality" of andropause and 60 percent of them are over the age of 65, according to Dr. Robert S. Tan, author of *The Andropause Mystery:*

Unraveling the Truths about Male Menopause. As men age, they lose hormones just as women do. When this happens to women it's referred to as menopause, whereas when this happens to men, it's known as andropause.

For women, menopause marks the end of the menstruation cycle. Although men have no visible signs of andropause, they just know because they feel differently, and because they feel differently, they act differently. Physical, mental and emotional changes are associated with andropause and each change tends to emerge gradually. As the level of testosterone drops in men, what little testosterone is left changes into estrogen. Aromatization (changing from one hormone to another) leaves men and women with higher levels of some hormones than others.

During menopause, women complain about hot flashes, depression, night sweats, mood swings and a loss in sexual desire. Once men have reached the andropause stage, men may experience similar symptoms.

> **Did you know?**
>
> - Most men will have lost 15 pounds of muscle by 40.
> - Between 40 and 60, the average man will lose more than 15 percent of bone.
> - 50 percent of the American male population will experience erectile dysfunction in their life.

Mr. or Mrs. Testosterone?

Testosterone is well known for its role in male puberty. After all, it promotes the growth of the reproductive tract, increases the length and diameter of the penis, helps in the development of the prostate and scrotum, and the sprouting of pubic and facial hair. Because of this, most people tend to think of testosterone as a "he" hormone in the same way that estrogen is thought of as a "she" hormone. However, as it turns out, men and women produce exactly the same hormones, only in different amounts. Men's bodies generate more than 10 milligrams of testosterone per day, 20 times more than women (an average of 1 milligram per day).

It's not unusual for a young woman in her prime (about 25) to have more testosterone than a man in his 60s. The tremendous amount of estrogen she possesses at the same time is what defines her as a woman. Furthermore, the estrogen balances the testosterone in her body and gives her stamina and endurance.

As women age, their levels of testosterone gradually declines. Women can especially feel this effect around menopause, when they also experience a precipitous drop in estrogen. The symptoms of a testosterone deficiency can include a loss of vital energy and feeling of well-being, a loss of familiar levels of sexual libido, sensitivity of nipples and genitals, a thinning of pubic hair, a lack confidence and depression. Women may also experience a "flatness" of mood, dry skin, brittle scalp hair, and loss of muscle tone and strength. It's understood that testosterone also contributes to the health of a woman's vulva, re-grows the vital tissue of the clitoris, and can play a role in curbing osteoporosis by helping maintain the density of our bones. Testosterone can also influence our cognitive function (memory, logic, etc.) as well.

Sexual Healing Time

Whether you are a man or a woman, your testosterone levels ultimately play a role in your desire for sexual activity. Although estrogen can also have a libido-enhancing effect, testosterone's effect is far greater. Over the years, researchers have found that testosterone levels influence a person's tendency towards aggression, cognition, sexuality and sex roles, occupation, personality, emotions, competitiveness, childhood behavior, facial expressions, disturbed relationships and more. Sexuality and libido are affected by much more than our biology. We can also add to the list-- stress, boredom, anxiety, disinterest and exhaustion.

Researchers agree that an annihilation of sexual desire can result from a significant reduction in testosterone. In both men and women, clinical studies show a greater correlation than was previously thought on the level of free and active testosterone and sexual activity. There appears to be a correlation between the ability to reach orgasm and a combination of higher DHEA and testosterone.

For men, sexual activity as well as erectile dysfunction becomes apparent as the level of testosterone declines past the age of 30. During the years when testosterone levels are at their peak, sexual activity is measured

TOP 11 REASONS FOR LOW TESTOSTERONE LEVELS

1) Menopause
2) Childbirth
3) Chemotherapy
4) Birth Control Pills
5) Adrenal Fatigue
6) Endometriosis
7) Depression
8) Severe Stress
9) Surgical Menopause
10) Anti-Cholesterol medication
11) Anti-Androgen medication

by the number of sexual intercourse encounters a person has. For example, a healthy 25-year-old who is in a relationship generally has sex three to four times per week. As testosterone levels drop, the number of times we have sex drops to about half, which means at 50 you're lucky if you have sex once a week.

With a loss in testosterone levels, there is a lack of sexual desire in both men and women. Men develop the "roving eye syndrome," while women enter the "no-man" zone.

"Love is a matter of chemistry, but sex is a matter of physics." ~Author Unknown

You Better Watch Your Step!!

If you find yourself tripping over dog toys, imaginary people, or your own feet more than you used to, most likely your testosterone levels are dropping.

Testosterone deficiencies cause both men and women to complain of losing depth perception. Many of my friends and patients have griped about how clumsy they've become. They're really not getting clumsier; they're losing their balance because of poor depth perception. They trip, fall off stairs, fumble over their feet and are constantly bumping into objects. On one occasion, a friend of mine whom I've known since med school told me he apologized to a store mannequin after he had bumped into her (it). He was convinced it was a person even after he had turned around. I couldn't contain myself; I had to laugh, even though I knew it wasn't very nice.

As in my friend's case, this is what happens when you lose testosterone. You don't know where you're going, and you might think that something is wrong with your eyes. While your eyesight could be dwindling, most likely it's not though. Your sense of perception has become fuddled; this is primarily because nerve electrical charges to muscle reaction time are much slower. As muscle reaction time becomes slower and slower, you continue to lose testosterone.

Keep in mind that in one way or another, testosterone affects all of the organs and systems in your body, which includes your cardiovascular health, the elasticity of your blood vessels, and the production of nitric oxide, a powerful compound that regulates your overall health.

One Size Doesn't Fit All

Just because everyone's body requires testosterone doesn't mean that everyone requires the same amount of the hormone. A person's body type dictates how much testosterone supplementation they will need. For example, a larger, more muscular individual will require more testosterone than a person with a smaller build. Interestingly, the same applies for hair growth. Men with a darker beard and denser body hair growth will require more testosterone than men who have less hair or thinner hair. Women who have a larger muscle distribution and wider hair distribution will also require more testosterone than a smaller woman with less hair. Experienced physicians can usually tell how much testosterone a patient may need by looking at their physical characteristics.

Are You a Candidate for Testosterone Supplementation?

If symptoms, signs, or your age cause you to suspect that you may have a testosterone deficiency, then your physician may perform a blood, urine or, more practically, a saliva testosterone test to evaluate the present level of your testosterone. If test results indicate that you do in fact have a testosterone loss, your physician or health worker may consider putting you on a supplemental testosterone program.

> **TRANSDERMAL APPLICATION HINT**
>
> Unless you like having certain parts of your body hairier and scarier than other parts, avoid applying Testosterone transdermal cream in the same area--be sure to rotate your application areas!!

Supplementation via bioidentical testosterone usually involves beginning with a smaller dose and then gradually increasing the amount that is needed to create a balance between testosterone and your other hormones. Another option your physician may take is to place you on an herbal extraction program, which consists of herbal extractions that act as secretagogues that convert into testosterone via a natural biochemical process. Bioidentical replacement therapy programs are crucial at any age for both men and women suffering from a testosterone deficiency. I can't stress it enough—don't put it off! If you are showing signs of testosterone loss, get your levels checked early—don't wait until your tank is completely empty!!!

Oral Testosterone Supplementation

If you are taking testosterone hormone supplements orally, then be sure to proceed with caution. When taken orally, hormones are absorbed through the GI tract and through mesenteric arteries. The liver then processes and metabolizes it. Being the main filter, the liver will automatically create sex hormone binding globulin (SHBG) to neutralize incoming excessive testosterone; therefore the increased level of SHBG will bind and neutralize the testosterone the individual has taken. Therefore, your net gain will actually be a big fat ZERO!

Testosterone Checklist	
You may have a Testosterone deficiency if you answer yes to any of these questions:	**You may have an excess of Testosterone if you answer yes to any of these questions:**
❑ Are your muscles weak and flabby? ❑ Do you have low self-esteem? ❑ Are you losing your muscle mass? ❑ Are you lacking in energy and stamina? ❑ Does your coordination and balance seem to be off? ❑ Are you mentally fatigued? ❑ Do you lack confidence? ❑ Do you have a decreased libido? ❑ Do you have trouble with orgasms or your sex drive? ❑ Are you gaining weight? ❑ Is your hair thinning? ❑ Do you feel depressed? ❑ Are you fatigued? ❑ Do you feel shriveled up and/or overly dry?	❑ Are you acting too aggressive or too pushy? ❑ Do you feel anxious or agitated? ❑ Are you over-confident? ❑ Are you experiencing acne eruptions? ❑ Do you have increased facial hair? ❑ Are you always angry? ❑ Do you have decreased HDL levels? ❑ Are your menstrual periods irregular?
If supplementation has already been taken, *increase* your dosage if you experience the above symptoms.	If supplementation has already been taken, *decrease* your dosage if you experience the above symptoms.

Injections

A common method (but not my favorite) for bioidentical testosterone supplementation is via injections. Typically, patients are given one injection per week, every two weeks, or monthly. Injections will usually last anywhere from two weeks to a month. Oftentimes with injections, the body receives a high level of testosterone that it isn't accustomed to. This in turn may cause unwanted side effects.

Transdermal

As with other hormone supplements, I strongly suggest using a transdermal form of bioidentical testosterone. Through liposome technology, testosterone is microencapsulated and can be rubbed on soft areas of the body like on the inside of your arm, behind your knee, or on the inner portion of your thighs. Apply the cream to the largest area of skin and rub vigorously until it's gone.

© Dr. Tai's Beauty Secret ©

Like all hormones, testosterone is produced in spurts throughout the day or approximately every two hours. Therefore, taking small amounts of transdermal testosterone daily is much closer to what our bodies would normally produce and it's absorbed slowly throughout the day into your body.

When using creams, lotions and gels, there are fewer side effects than there are with injections or tablets. Oftentimes, men apply creams on their chest; older men (60+) should do this especially if they see their breast size is increasing.

For women who wish to avoid testosterone's side effects, they should use natural transdermal estrogen as a balancer. This allows the potential side effects of testosterone to be neutralized. Side effects of testosterone can include over-aggressiveness or bossy behavior, a bad temper, insensitivity, acne formation, the feeling of being over-sexed, and facial hair growth on both men and women. Additional and more severe side-effects include insomnia, heat intolerance and the possibility of tachycardia and arrhythmia (irregular heartbeat rhythm). Should you experience these effects, decrease your dosages to half and wait two weeks. If side effects still occur, reduce to half of that half again, and keep reducing until all symptoms disappear.

CHAPTER 18

Progesterone--a woman's personal bodyguard

"They call it PMS because Mad Cow Disease was already taken."

~Author Unknown

Just as it is a man's duty to protect women; the hormone progesterone protects women in a very important way. In the past, estrogen has always been considered to be a woman's Number 1 sex hormone. However, progesterone should be considered a close second. After all, it's progesterone that helps to keep a woman's body out of trouble.

As I've mentioned before, hormones have a profound effect on your everyday health and wellbeing. Hormones affect every cell within your body. Not only do hormones have individual effects, they also interact with each other to produce dramatic effects in the body. For example, women need estrogen, but sometimes the body produces too much of it, and they need a balancer such as progesterone to keep the body from going haywire. It's hard to be beautiful when your body is on the fritz.

Did you know?

Too much estrogen can stir up a multitude of metabolic disturbances. Progesterone, on the other hand, has a balancing effect that prevents an excess of estrogen from being toxic and harmful to health.

Where does progesterone come from?

Progesterone is made in the ovaries of menstruating women and by the placenta during pregnancy. About 20 to 25 mg of progesterone are produced per day during a woman's monthly cycle and up to 300 to 400 mg are produced daily during pregnancy. Progesterone is a precursor to many steroid hormones and performs a myriad of different functions.

PMS, periods, and progesterone

Almost all women have experienced symptoms of PMS, which frequently occurs in the second half of the menstrual period. Estrogen dominance has created an imbalance where there isn't enough progesterone available to balance out the estrogen. Symptoms of excess estrogen depend on the individual and include moodiness, abdominal cramps, headaches, etc.

Eighty percent of women suffer from PMS, and as it increases in severity, women report having an increased appetite, food cravings and fatigue. While excess estrogen interferes with thyroid function, progesterone improves the thyroid hormone. Estrogen interference occurs because the production of the thyroid binding globulin is accelerate, which makes for less free and available thyroid to be used by the body. This is yet one more way that progesterone works hard every day to protect a woman's overall health.

Women's love/hate relationship with periods

It's not unusual for women to lose roughly 3 to 5 ounces of blood during their menstrual cycles. Some months bring a heavier flow than other months. Because of their inconvenience and unpredictable nature, most women do not have a loving relationship with their periods.

Although most women don't consider their periods to be very beneficial, periods are actually supposed to be a welcomed relief. Not only is the woman releasing ovum (eggs), it's her body's way of eliminating unwanted substances. While men can release environmental toxins via their urinary system, respiratory system, skin and gastrointestinal system, women have the natural advantage of having their periods. Just as trees and plants purify the air we breathe, periods do a remarkable job of purifying a woman's body from pesticides and pollutants.

Menstruation 101

On average, menstrual cycles last 28-days and five major hormones are involved in creating a cycle: gonadotropin releasing hormone (GNRH), follicle stimulating hormone (FSH), luteinizing hormone (LH), estrogen, and progesterone.

MENSTRUAL CYCLE- STAGE I

During the first stage of a menstrual cycle, estrogen dominates the period from day 1 to day 14, or the first day your period begins until seven days after your period ends.

MENSTRUAL CYCLE- STAGE 2

The second phase, from day 14 until day 28, is known as the luteonizing phase of the menstrual period.

If the egg isn't fertilized and implanted by this time, progesterone levels diminish and dramatically drop. This means that a woman has approximately 20-50 pg/ml* of progesterone. At the highest point of the luteonizing phase, it can be is as high as 250 pg/ml (as measured on the saliva test).

MENSTRUAL CYCLE- STAGE 3

Progesterone levels are highest during pregnancy. The progesterone count in a pregnant woman's saliva can be as high as 2200 pg/ml.

Shortly after the birth of a baby, progesterone levels will return to a normal 50 pg/ml. To a woman's body—dropping from 2200 pg/ml to 50 pg/ml—is a radical change that can cause potential problems.

At the post-partum stage, mothers can experience depression, anxiety, and excruciating headaches.

Women ask, we tell

EXCESS ESTROGEN

- Why do women gain weight before their monthly periods?   ~Olivia, 27

Shortly before a woman's period, her progesterone level decreases, leading to symptoms of excess estrogen. Surplus estrogen causes fluid retention, sometimes increasing body weight by approximately five pounds. Based on their poor eating habits and PMS cravings, women end up gaining even more weight. Bringing progesterone and estrogen in balance with each other can work as a natural diuretic to help maintain weight levels even while a woman is on her period.

An amazing, but little-known quality of progesterone is that it possesses the *diuretic effect*, or the ability of ridding of excess water in the body. At the appropriate levels, progesterone has the capability to remove excess water from tissues, decreasing swelling and bloating effects that most women experience during menstruation. In addition, progesterone is known to lower blood pressure and significantly improve the vascular tone.

CYSTS AND FIBROIDS

- Why do I continue to get cysts on my breast and how can I prevent getting more?
  ~Peyton, 36

One thing that estrogen is good at is stimulating breast cell growth, which possibly leads to cystic changes of the breast as well as uterine and ovarian fibroids. Estrogen causes multiple changes in the breast, fibroid changes of the uterus, and polycystic and multi-cystic changes of the ovaries. All of these problems typically require women to seek treatment.

Increasing your intake of bioidentical progesterone will allow you to decrease the occurrence of fibroids, cysts and tumorous growths on soft tissues like your breasts, uterus and ovaries. Progesterone controls and regulates cell multiplication. When progesterone is properly balanced within the breast tissues, the hormone actually prevents and diminishes the occurrence of breast cysts, fibroids and tumors.

Hormones out of whack!

Typical complaints heard from female patients include weight gain, fatigue, libido loss, depression, headaches, joint pain and mood swings. Other common problems include uterine fibroids, cancer, fibrocystic breast disease, menstrual problems, autoimmune disorders, pre-menopausal bone loss and a high incidence of osteoporosis after menopause. As a result, physicians and scientists are becoming increasingly aware of a common link between these symptoms and diseases and an imbalance between progesterone and estrogen-- the primary female sex hormones.

> **Sound familiar?**
>
> If you seem to be consistently nervous, anxious, and fearful and depressed, you may have a progesterone deficiency.
>
> If this seems like you, try bioidentical progesterone as a natural sedative.

It is essential that these two hormones are in balance within a woman's body. At different times throughout a woman's life, such factors as stress, obesity, poor liver function, birth control pills, plant estrogens (soy, flaxseeds, red clover), hormone replacement therapy, perimenopause, and glandular dysfunction can cause hormonal imbalance.

Regardless of the cause, the end result of an imbalance between estrogen and progesterone equals a condition that researcher, Dr. John Lee has termed "estrogen dominance." This condition can result in symptoms of PMS, perimenopause, or menopause. (Lee, J.R., What Your Doctor May Not Tell You About Menopause. Warner Books, May, 1996).

ENDOMETRIOSIS

Another consequence to having an imbalance between estrogen and progesterone is *endometriosis*. Due to exceedingly high levels of estrogen in the early part of the menstrual period--predominantly in the inner lining of the uterus-- a thickening of blood supply is more than likely to occur.

Endometriosis causes blood to become darker. Instead of a bright, crimson red, blood turns a dark burgundy, almost brown like chocolate syrup. Women who suffer with endometriosis often experience increased damage to their ovarian tubes. This painful and sometimes dangerous condition (i.e., hemorrhaging) can be prevented simply by balancing estrogen levels with progesterone.

Endometriosis, which is diagnosed by gynecologists around the world, commonly treats the condition with *synthetic progesterone* known as *progestins.*

Usually, during the beginning stages of progesterone supplementation, patients may experience a bleeding surge. However, this is a normal—it only means that the progesterone is ridding the body of old blood, or blood that's been left behind from a previous period.

Good for your brain

Have you ever thought you were losing your mind or going crazy? Higher progesterone levels can play a significant role in regenerating and protecting the neuron cells of the brain. This allows for a healthier cellular brain as well as improving memory and sharpness of thinking. Progesterone not only has a direct effect of neural functions—it also it moderates sugar metabolism as it increases the oxygenation of the brain and the rest of the tissues of the body.

"Body and mind, like man and wife, do not always agree to die together." ~Charles Caleb Colton

Make no bones about it!!

It is a widely known fact that estrogen is essential for healthy bones, and that when estrogen production is reduced, as normally occurs in postmenopausal women and after exposure to radiation or chemotherapeutic drugs, bones become brittle and break easily. Recent studies indicate that bioidentical progesterone also plays a key role protecting bone health.

In 1990, Dr. John R. Lee, a renowned physician from California, conducted a three-year study with 100 post-menopausal patients aged 40 to 80. Dr. Lee noted that 63 of his study's participants, who had regular supplementation of progesterone, had an increase of bone mineralization by 15.4 percent. From his study, Dr. Lee concluded that by using transdermal bioidentical progesterone, the osteoporatic rate upon which bones demineralize can be delayed. (Lee, J.R. "Osteoporosis reversal with transdermal progesterone." *Lancet*, 1990; 336:1327.)

That same year, Dr. Jeri Lynn Prior at the University of British Columbia found that progesterone aided in the formation and maintenance of bones, as it was able to speed growth and healing rates.

Five years later, the PEPI trials (Postmenopausal Estrogen Progestin Interventions), one of the largest studies to have ever been conducted on progesterone, tracked 875 women aged 45 to 64 for approximately three years.

The Power of Natural Progesterone *(La M., Natural Woman, Natural Menopause, NY:HarperCollins, 1997)*

1. Balances estrogen
2. No accumulation in body
3. Improves sleep
4. Naturally calms the body
5. Improves high blood pressure
6. Enhances burning of body fats
7. Lowers cholesterol
8. May Protects from breast cancer
9. Enhances growth of scalp hair
10. Improves libido
11. Helps to prevent hardening of the arteries.

The researchers of this major study concluded that bioidentical estrogen, combined with bioidentical progesterone, had the most effect on raising HDL ("good" cholesterol) without producing the pre-cancerous uterine effects that synthetic forms of estrogen and progesterone tend to bring about. The PEPI trials clearly demonstrated that natural progesterone works better than progestin (synthetic progesterone) in protecting the heart and uterus.

Heart Health

Another fascinating attribute of progesterone is the ability to prevent a condition known as thrombophlebitis or moving blood clots. The condition is as scary as its name. It's when clots form on your leg's veins (as well as other deep veins), then breaks away and migrates to your heart! In addition to having ugly legs that look like a road map with a bunch of blue and purple squiggly lines, this condition is not healthy.

An excess of synthetic estrogen can create thrombophlebitis, however, progesterone can moderate the excess effects that cause it. Progesterone also improves the spasticity of the heart's many blood vessels.

Throughout the duration of menopause, many women can develop atherosclerosis, a condition when patients frequently suffer from severe spasms from contractions in the heart's muscles. Progesterone can relieve the body from producing fatal myocardial infarctions or deadly heart spasms so that your heart can continue beating.

"I have found that synthetic progestins can lead to serious cardiac side effects in my patients, including shortness of breath, fatigue, chest pain, and high blood pressure," says Dr. Stephen Sinatra, cardiologist. (Sinatra, S. *Heart Sense for Women*. Washington DC: Lifeline Press, 2000)

Progesterone for men

Like estrogen, progesterone is commonly thought of as a 'female' sex hormone. This belief is misleading as it is vital to sustain not just health but life itself in ALL mammals of both sexes.

It's inevitable that men will lose testosterone as their body's age. Testosterone is converted into dihydrotestosterone (DHT), which some believe is the cause of benign prostatic hyperplasia (BPH) and cancer. Progesterone's main effect in men is the ability to be converted into testosterone.

Reasons why men should supplement their progesterone levels:

- It provides a basis for testosterone conversion.
- It occupies estrogen receptor sites in the prostate in order to avoid complications such as the development of prostate cancer.

As it moves throughout a man's body, progesterone snatches estrogen cells from receptor sites. Therefore, keeping receptor sites busy with a lot of progesterone can prevent estrogen from causing damage to the tissues.

Because estrogen causes the cells of these tissues to reproduce and multiply at an accelerated rate, these tissues become hypertrophied, or enlarged, which is exactly how benign tumors grow on tissue sites.

Prostate health

Men with sufficient progesterone levels are less likely to experience enlarged prostates, a problem effecting more than 35 million men in the U.S. A progesterone deficiency can make urinating painful and potentially cancerous.

If enough progesterone is present, the progesterone hormone occupying the same receptor sites will moderate and diminish the production of the excess tissue created by estrogen.

As men and women age, aromatization increases the production of testosterone to estrogen, or the production of estrogen from fat tissue. For men, testosterone is converted into estrogen. If we can use progesterone to occupy the receptor sites in the prostate, we can decrease estrogen's effects on the prostate. If the progesterone hormone is occupying those receptor sites, there's a greater likelihood that excess estrogen won't damage prostate tissue and lead to tumorous growths.

SO, WHAT HAVE WE LEARNED ABOUT PROGESTERONE?

- Progesterone is the primary hormone of fertility and pregnancy. It is essential to the survival of the fertilized egg, then the embryo, then the fetus. In pregnancy, it prevents the shedding of the uterine lining, as a drop in progesterone can result in a miscarriage.

- Natural progesterone helps to counter balance the negative effects of estrogen. When there is not enough progesterone to counterbalance estrogen, one may begin to have symptoms of "estrogen dominance". For example: severe PMS, heavy or irregular periods, irritability, weight gain, anxiety, hair loss, low libido, fibrocystic breasts, endometriosis, and uterine fibroids, to name a few.

Synthetic vs. bioidentical progesterone

Medroxy progesterone acetate, or MPA, is synthetic progesterone and belongs to the *progestin* class of drugs. Chemically modified, MPA isn't at all compatible to the progesterone the body produces and isn't even remotely similar to the bioidentical form of progesterone. Progestin (synthetic progesterone) side effects include bloating, nausea and depression. Natural progesterone eliminated these side effects. *(American Family Physicians, 1999; 16(1): 264)*

While pharmaceutical companies want you to believe that MPA is similar to natural progesterone, it may have only an 8 percent biologic activity similar to natural progesterone. Over 90 percent of synthetic progesterone is foreign to the body and our tissue receptor sites. When obtained from plant sources, progesterone has fewer side effects when compared to synthetic progestins. *(American Family Physicians, 2000; 62(8):1839)*

You may have a progesterone deficiency if you have:	You may have a progesterone excess if you have:
<ul><li>Severe PMS symptoms</li><li>Depression or mood swings</li><li>Anxiety, nervousness, or irritability</li><li>Breast swelling</li><li>Bloating or water retention</li><li>Bone loss/osteoporosis</li><li>Uterine fibroids</li><li>Excessive menstrual bleeding</li><li>Decreased HDL</li><li>Insomnia</li></ul>	<ul><li>Hot flashes</li><li>Increased cortisol</li><li>Decreased glucose tolerance</li><li>Increased fat storage</li><li>Increased appetite / carb cravings</li><li>Depression</li><li>A drunk feeling</li><li>Water retention caused by progesterone supplementation</li><li>Drowsiness</li></ul>
If you already use a progesterone supplement, **increase** your dosage if you checked any of the above symptoms.	If you already use a progesterone supplement, **decrease** your dosage if you checked any of the above symptoms.

ॐ Dr. Tai's Amazing Beauty Secret ॐ

For women with severe PMS symptoms such as mood swings, anxiety attacks, and depression, have your saliva analyzed for progesterone--specifically from the 21st to the 28th day of your cycle. In relationship to estrogen levels during that time, most PMS symptoms occur near the period. PMS relief can be found by using transdermal liposome progesterone when applied throughout the body from day 14-28, or the first day of bleeding, whichever comes first.

For most menopausal women, the optimum plan requires you to follow just two simple instructions. First, test your progesterone levels via a saliva hormone test. Second, with the assistance of a doctor, use supplemental progesterone on the upper torso, around the breasts, all over your chest, making your way down to your tummy. Make sure the cream is spread widely across your skin—working the cream vigorously into the skin will generate a good circulation. This will assure the largest spreading of progesterone throughout the body and prevent a concentration of the hormone in one small area. Start the supplementation on day 7 of your cycle, and continue with 20 mg in the evening and 20 mg in the morning from day 7 to day 28. Discontinue supplementation from day 1 to day 7.

It doesn't matter whether you have your menstrual period—you still should discontinue supplementation on day 28 and stop supplementation for 5-7 days. Occasionally, we see individuals who choose to supplement every day without taking a five-day break, but as always, that should be completely up to their doctor. I've heard of no harm done to patients that haven't discontinued supplementation, so it's only advised to give your body a break. Follow nature and do what you feel. However, please ask your doctor prior to starting supplementation.
H

CHAPTER 19

Melatonin

"When you have insomnia, you're never really asleep, and you're never really awake."
~From the movie *Fight Club*, based on the novel by Chuck Palahniuk

One would think that getting a good night's rest would be an easy thing to do seeing how sleeping is a natural physiological function of the body. Unfortunately, sleeping is becoming harder for many people to do, especially as they get older. So why is this? The level of *melatonin* within our body decreases as we age. In addition, with the onset of menopause comes a severe decline in melatonin secretion. *(Lieberman, S., The Real Vitamin and Mineral Book. Avery Publ. 1997.p.216)*

Why Can't I Sleep?

If you find yourself tossing and turning every night, chances are it's because your body is having trouble producing a sufficient amount of melatonin.

Melatonin controls the body's "circadian cycle," an internal 24-hour time-keeping system that plays an important role in when we fall asleep and when we wake up.

Melatonin is produced when the amino acid *tryptophan* converts enzymes. It's worth noting that stress depletes tryptophan. You need tryptophan along with vitamin B complex to convert tryptophan into melatonin.

So during stressful times, tryptophan depletion leads to a reduction in melatonin, and melatonin is one of the few hormones that actually lowers cortisol levels to help you stay cool, calm, and collected when life gets crazy.

Where Does Melatonin Come From?

Created by the pineal (say peen-ee-al) gland, melatonin is the hormone responsible for the "circadian cycle," or the sleep/wake cycle. The *pineal gland*, which resembles a pea or a kernel of corn, is a tiny gland in the center of the brain.

Although it is situated deep within the brain and doesn't have access to light, the pineal gland does contain light-sensitive cells. When light enters the eyes, it travels to the retina.

From the retina, a message is sent through the optic nerve to the hypothalamus (a much bigger gland than the pineal) and that's when the pineal is informed whether light is present or not. Scientists used to think the pineal was as useless as a person's pinky finger, but without the tiny organ, the body wouldn't have any melatonin, which is a modulating hormone that relaxes us and tells us when it's time to rest.

How much sleep do we really need?

Melatonin Facts

- Improves mood
- Helps stress respons
- Assists immune system function
- Stimulates release (sex hormones
- Have powerful antioxidant effect

Bland J., "Obesity an endocrine signaling." Health Comm International, Inc. 1999, p.124.

The amount of sleep needed varies from person to person. Generally speaking, most healthy adults are programmed for 16 hours of wakefulness and need an average of eight hours of sleep a night.

Some individuals can function without sleepiness or drowsiness after as little as six hours of sleep. Others can't perform at their peak until they've slept at least ten hours. And, contrary to common myth, the need for sleep doesn't decline with age but it may become harder to sleep for six to eight hours at one time.
(Van Dongen & Dinges, Principles & Practice of Sleep Medicine, 2000)

Always listen to Mom!

Do you remember your mother ever telling you that if you didn't get to sleep, you wouldn't grow? Well, she was right. She wasn't pulling your leg. Sleeping does help children grow. As a matter of fact, children grow as they sleep.

During the adolescent stage, melatonin blood levels reach a new high. These surging levels of melatonin tell the pituitary gland to produce a luteinizing hormone (LH) and follicle-stimulating hormone (FSH) when puberty begins. It's all downhill from there, because after puberty, melatonin production begins to decline. This is the reason your teenager would prefer to sleep until noon and your eldest neighbors are up at the crack of dawn power-walking.

By age 60, we produce half the amount of melatonin we produced in our 20s. Once we lose the ability to produce proper amounts of melatonin, it is more difficult to fall asleep than it is to wake up.

Are you dead or alive?

As Americans become more and more focused on working to put food on the table and gas in their car, sleeping becomes less of a priority. Many think, "Why should I sleep for eight hours when I should be working and making money?" Well, because, if you didn't sleep, you would be digging an early grave for yourself. The human body can only go so long without sleep.

In a study conducted by researcher Alan Rechtshaffen, rats died after two weeks of sleep deprivation. Although no deaths were reported from sleep deprivation in humans, at most, people can tolerate going 11 days without sleep. Not only will you feel like dying without sleep, you'll also look like death. Rechtshaffen also found that the skin, the body's largest organ, suffers most from sleep deprivation.

> **Did you know?**
>
> Sleeping pills can be addictive and can also cause a "hang-over effect"

Once you start popping, there's no stopping!!

Temporary sleep relief is habit-forming and can leave you feeling groggy in the morning and unsatisfied at the amount of sleep you received the night before. Sadly, sleep, which is a physiologically normal function as important as eating, drinking and having sex, is being managed by a multitude of drugs. Sure, sleep sedatives will help for a few nights, but they'll also cause a variety of health problems along the way like raising your blood pressure.

What causes melatonin levels to decrease?	
Tobacco adrenergic blockers	Alpha
Electromagnetic fields	Alcohol
Caffeine blockers	Beta
Tranquilizers	Aspirin
Ibuprofen channel blockers	Calcium

Functions of Melatonin

1) Induces sleep
2) Improves mood
3) Helps stress response
4) Assists immune system function
5) Stimulates release of sex hormones
6) Has powerful antioxidant effects (Bland J., "Obesity and endocrine signaling." Health Comm International, Inc. 1999, p.124.)
7) Helps prevent cancer
8) Blocks estrogen binding to receptors. (Lieberman, S., The Real Vitamin and Mineral Book. Avery Publ. 1997,.p.216)
9) Stimulates parathyroid bone formation. (Lieberman, S., The Real Vitamin and Mineral Book.

Avery Publ. 1997.p.216)
10)   Production of growth hormone
11)   Decreases and modulates cortisol

Helen's Story

Years ago, I had a neighbor, Helen, who was a lawyer. She was a rather petite woman. At that time, Helen was no older than 40, yet she appeared to be much older; she rarely looked anyone in the eye and she never smiled. She looked rough...real rough. In fact, she reminded me more of an inmate who had been doing hard time for the last 20 years rather than the prominent attorney that she was. Her hair was boldly streaked with grey and she had deeply embedded facial wrinkles. She had bruises around her once beautiful blue eyes—now they were merely two dark circles outlined by a pair of tortoise-shell eyeglasses.

Helen told me that she hadn't slept in days, and because she hadn't slept in days, her performance in the courtroom suffered. To overcome her sleep problems, Helen had taken all sorts of drastic measures just to fall asleep---sleeping pills, sedatives and frequently overdosing on Nyquil.

I explained to Helen that her melatonin levels were decreasing at an above-average rate and that she somehow needed to replenish her lost hormones. Well...Helen was a good lawyer and did her research. She replenished her lost melatonin levels by using a bioidentical form of melatonin: a supplement which consisted of a whole family of different antioxidants and an alpha lipoic acid called Antioxidant Specialist.

I felt guilty for thinking she was a rude, anti-social woman who would only talk to people if they'd pay her to talk for them. She wasn't—in fact, Helen was simply misunderstood because she was always tired. Once she started sleeping peacefully she became an entirely different person—like the difference between night and day. Not only did her eyes come back to life, her skin radiated beauty and her attitude shined.

Moral of Helen's story

Natural medicine is much more effective than any sort of pharmaceutically compounded prescription.

What causes melatonin levels to increase?

- Supplementation
- Darkness
- Sleep
- Exercise

DOES THIS SOUND LIKE YOU?	
You may have a melatonin deficiency if you have:	You may have a melatonin excess if you have:
❑ Insomnia ❑ The inability to stay asleep ❑ Waking periodically throughout the night ❑ Jet lag ❑ Difficulty adjusting to time zones	❑ Inability to wake ❑ Sleepy/ groggy after waking ❑ Reoccurring nightmares or unpleasant dreams ❑ Daytime sleepiness / fatigue ❑ Suppressed serotonin ❑ Suppressed craving for sugar ❑ Increased cortisol and fat ❑ Headaches
If you already use a melatonin supplement, **increase** your dosage if you checked any of the above symptoms.	If you already use a melatonin supplement, **decrease** your dosage if you checked any of the above symptoms

---

ও DR. TAI'S AMAZING BEAUTY SECRET ও

People who sleep more lower their levels of stress; so for those of you who are passionate about getting ahead and being successful, do it by getting a little more "R&R."

By taking bioidentical melatonin, I am confident that you will fall asleep quicker and feel much more rested in the morning.

I used to have a terrible time falling asleep, and out of all the supplements I've used, melatonin has never failed me. It's been two years since I've started taking melatonin and I've developed so much energy because I sleep straight through the night instead of waking up at irregular intervals as I once used to.

Ever since I started taking melatonin my dreams and days have become sweeter than ever!

CHAPTER 20

Thyroid: the little gland with a big job

"In order to change, we must be sick and tired of being sick and tired." ~Author Unknown

Does your body feel broken and ugly? Do you find yourself balding or losing hair? Are you always tired and have trouble concentrating or remembering things? Have you experienced an unexplained weight gain or are you having problems losing weight regardless of what you do?

While some people assume that the above symptoms are normal signs of aging, the truth is---they aren't!! While our bodies do exhibit some changes as we get older, we shouldn't assume that all changes are normal. You could very possibly be suffering from a thyroid problem. Thyroid disorders can cause serious problems and shouldn't be overlooked or written off as mere signs of aging.

What is the thyroid?

The thyroid is a small gland, shaped like a butterfly, in the lower part of your neck. The purpose of the thyroid gland is to produce, collect, and secrete thyroid hormones into your bloodstream. Two main hormones released by the thyroid are triiodothyronine (T3) and thyroxine (T4). These hormones, T3 and T4, affect almost every cell in your body and help control your body's metabolism. Thyroid cells gather circulating iodine from the blood to create T3 and T4, which are then released into the bloodstream and carried to organs in the body, including the liver, kidneys, muscles, heart, and brain.

Although it weighs less than an ounce, the thyroid gland has an enormous effect on your health. The thyroid hormones regulate all aspects of your metabolism--from the rate at which your heart beats to how quickly you burn calories. Other vital body functions affected by the thyroid include: the respiratory rate, skin maintenance, growth, heat production, fertility and digestion.

How does the thyroid work?

Thyroid hormones influence the metabolic rate in two ways: by stimulating almost every tissue in the body to produce proteins and by increasing the amount of oxygen that cells use.

T4, the major hormone produced by the thyroid gland, has only a minimal effect on boosting the body's metabolic rate. Instead, T4 is converted into T3, the more active hormone. The conversion of T4 to T3 occurs in the liver and other tissues. The body's momentary needs as well as the presence of certain illnesses direct the conversion of T4 to T3.

In order to produce thyroid hormones, the thyroid gland requires iodine, an element commonly found in food and water. The thyroid gland captures iodine and processes it into thyroid hormones. As thyroid hormones are expended, a small amount of the iodine contained in the hormones is released, and then returned to the thyroid gland, which is recycled to produce more thyroid hormones.

The T4 hormone, which regulates critical functions such as heart rate, digestion, physical growth, and mental development, comprises approximately 80 percent of the thyroid gland. A weak thyroid, which is the result of an inadequate amount of T4, can retard life-sustaining processes, damage organs and tissues throughout the body, and lead to life-threatening complications.

Thyroid Functions

- Controls carbohydrates, protein, and fat metabolism
- Directs proper utilization of vitamin
- Improves digestion
- Regulates mitochondria function(energy of the cells)
- Promotes muscle growth and repair
- Stimulates nerve activities
- Increases blood flow
- Improves overall body hormone excretion
- Increases amount of oxygen used by cells
- Modulates sexual function

Stop for a minute and....think!!!

Are you much heavier than you'd like to be? Have you become your own worst enemy? Do you find yourself moping around the house like a slug wearing baggy sweat pants and a holey t-shirt you haven't washed in a month? You only shower and wash your hair when your bodily stench becomes truly unbearable to the point your neighbors across the street can smell you. You're grouchy and eager to start the pettiest arguments with anyone, and really, who could blame you? You feel ugly and fat although you haven't eaten in days (if not, weeks). On average, you may only eat four or five meals a week. You intentionally leave your refrigerator and cupboards empty. You keep telling yourself that the less you eat, the more weight you'll lose. While this rationale might have worked when you were 20, you're now 45 and nothing is working. In fact, you feel like you're getting fatter just thinking about it.

If you think you resemble the person described in this scenario, it's very likely that you're one of the millions of people who suffer from *"hypothyroidism."*

HYPOTHYROID SYMPTOMS

- Lethargy and decreased energy
- Intolerance to coldness
- Tingling and numbness in extremities
- Muscle pain and stiffness
- Constipation
- Weight gain
- Dry, scaly or yellowish skin
- Coarse hair and skin
- Depression
- Forgetfulness
- Personality changes
- Anemia
- Prolonged or heavy menstrual cycles

Troubled thyroid

As long as your thyroid keeps producing the right amount of hormones, your metabolism continues to function normally. However, when the thyroid gland doesn't work properly, the fragile balance of thyroid hormones within your body is disturbed. If you have too little thyroid hormone in your blood, your body metabolism slows down, creating the condition called *"hypothyroidism."* If you have too much thyroid hormone in your blood, your body metabolism speeds up, creating a condition known as *"hyperthyroidism."*

Diagnosing thyroid problems

Detecting the clinical signs of hypothyroidism (under activity) and hyperthyroidism (over activity) can be perplexing. However, recognizing clinical symptoms are especially important in thyroid function conditions. Since blood tests TSH, T4 and T3 alone do not provide adequate information for complete diagnosis, tests may not always confirm the diagnosis. Auto-antibodies in the blood almost always test negative, and thyroid ultrasound studies are rare and uncommon (most clinics aren't equipped with this piece of equipment). These combined factors make testing for thyroid dysfunctions a complicated process.

Proteins in the blood carry thyroid hormones to such targets as the lungs, bones, heart, stomach, intestines, skin, hair, nails, and the brain. Because thyroid hormones are attached to proteins, less than one percent floats freely in a person's bloodstream.

If your doctor knows the total TSH and T4 amount in your blood, he or she needs to order a second test to determine the unbound T3 (the active hormones).

MENOPAUSE AND THE THYROID

Because ovaries have thyroid receptors and the thyroid gland has ovarian receptors, losing testosterone and Estradiol during menopause can cause lower thyroid function and production.

(Pamela, S. HRT, The Answers. Healthy Living Books. 2003)

GOOD FOR THE BRAIN

- In order to maintain optimal brain function, older patients may require middle to high level circulating thyroid.
- Hypothyroid patients may suffer subtle cognitive deficits.

(Journal of Gerontology: Medical Sciences, 1999; 54A (3): M111-M116)

The body's thermostat

To visualize how the thyroid gland works, think of it as a house's furnace and the pituitary gland as the thermostat that controls the temperature within the house. Thyroid hormones are like heat. When the heat circulates back to the thermostat, it turns the thermostat off. As the room cools (the thyroid hormone levels drop), the thermostat turns back on (TSH increases) and the furnace produces more heat (thyroid hormones). The pituitary gland itself is regulated by another gland, known as the hypothalamus. The hypothalamus is part of the brain and produces TSH-releasing hormone (TRH), which tells the pituitary gland to stimulate the thyroid gland (release TSH). One might imagine the hypothalamus as the person who sets the thermostat; since it tells the pituitary gland at what level the thyroid should be set.

The body's factory

Another way to think of the thyroid gland is like a factory. To produce its products (secretions), it must have raw material (iodine). If it lacks the necessary raw materials, the factory's production lags. When this happens, signals from elsewhere in the body may be sent telling the gland that it needs to increase its output. In an attempt to accommodate the request, the thyroid gland may get larger, but it simply cannot increase production because it lacks the necessary raw materials. The thyroid gland may continue to enlarge until a noticeable lump appears in the throat. This swelling--or "*goiter*"--may become large enough to interfere with breathing or swallowing. Goiters can be hereditary, sporadic, or endemic, but can also be caused due to a lack of sufficient iodine in the diet.

Importance of iodine

Iodine is vital for good thyroid function, which in turn is essential for health. Iodine deficiency during pregnancy and early infancy can result in cretinism (irreversible mental retardation and severe motor impairments). In adults, low iodine intake (or very high intake) can cause hypothyroidism.

Iodine affects different tissues in various ways. A 1995 study concluded that iodine improves ovarian and breast fibroids and cysts while sidestepping abnormal metabolisms and breast cancer. In iodine-deficient female rats, it was observed that iodine traveled into the chest cavity and rested within the breast tissues. When iodine and iodide were combined, benign growths in the rats decreased in size. (Erskin et al. "Iodine response in rates." *Biological Trace Element Research*, 1995; 49;209-219.)

> **Good to know**
>
> Excessive levels of various hormones (ex.-testosterone) can give you false thyroid hormone results. Synthetic estrogens increase the amount of thyroxin-binding proteins in your body, creating a greater number of unbound thyroid hormones.

The "Goiter Belt" of America

Endemic (continuously present in a specific community) goiters are usually caused by inadequate dietary intake of iodine in geographical areas with iodine-depleted soil such as areas away from the sea coast. The Great Lakes, Midwest, and Inter-mountain regions of the U.S. have been dubbed as the "goiter belt." Fortunately, iodine deficiency is now rare in the U.S. because of widespread distribution of foods from iodine-sufficient areas and the use of iodized table salt.

People who live on coastal regions have a greater advantage to the multiple sources of iodine found in seaweed and seafood. Asians, whose cultural diet is rich in seafood and seaweed, tend to have fewer thyroid problems than any other group.

Iodine is mostly found in fish, and to a lesser extent in milk, eggs, fruits and meat. To avoid severe thyroid problems or iodine deficiencies, 200 to 300 micrograms of iodine a day is necessary.

Because some regions of the world such as the valleys of the Alps and Pyrenees mountains, Syria, India, and China lack iodine in the land and water supplies, millions of people suffer from severe goiters, which have led to hearing and speech defects and, in more severe cases, cretinism.

HINTS FOR A HEALTHY THYROID

- Add a pinch of iodized salt daily with a well-balanced, nutritious meal.
- Take supplemental seaweed or concentrated iodine or iodide.

Selenium and the thyroid gland

In addition to iodine, selenium is an essential mineral for maintaining proper function of the thyroid gland. While selenium is necessary for the thyroid gland to produce the most active form of T3, it also helps regulate the amount of hormone that is produced.

Get your body moving!

Of course exercising is good for you, but did you know that it's great for maintaining a healthy thyroid? And I don't mean going to the gym and pumping iron until you pass out! In fact, over exercising can exhaust the adrenals, which can in turn negatively affect the thyroid. Over exercising exhausts the adrenals and the thyroid by causing weight to fluctuate. Rather than killing yourself with vigorous exercise, try moderate exercise such as a 20-minute jog in your neighborhood or a 30-minute walk in the park. Instead of driving, ride a bike; try to substitute convenience with body movement. The more activity, the better you'll feel. Exercise promotes a healthy self by improving heart and lung function while raising good cholesterol and strengthening muscles.

No excuses allowed!!

If you have hypothyroid and are trying to lose weight, you will no doubt be challenged as your energy levels will probably be lower than everyone else's. But you can't use your condition as an excuse to avoid exercise. Force yourself to exercise four to five times a week instead of three.

You'll need to make a concerted effort throughout your supplementation period to be as active as possible, especially under circumstances when sleeping sounds much more fun than exercising. Whatever you do, you need to get your heart pumping enough blood for a healthy respiratory and nervous system.

Now on the other hand, if you have hyperthyroid, I would highly suggest that you relax and exercise mildly until your thyroid problem has been treated. Hyperthyroid patients have above-average heartbeats, and exercising may cause even abnormally higher heartbeats. To be on the safe side and avoid having a heart attack, proceed with caution; treat your hyperthyroid and then get exercising!

Metabolism--functional or dysfunctional?

When we eat, food is converted into energy. The term "metabolism" actually refers to the way--not the speed--that our body processes and uses the food we eat. Rather than saying we have a fast or slow metabolism, it's more accurate to say our metabolism is efficient or functional versus inefficient or dysfunctional.

> **Heart Fact**
>
> Hypothyroidism is an indicator of atherosclerosis and myocardial infarction in elderly women **(Annals of Internal Medicine, 2000; 132: 270-8).**

Hyperthyroid and hypothyroid can both be differentiated by how fast or how slow a person loses weight. Most people with hypothyroid have trouble losing weight, while most people with hyperthyroid have trouble gaining weight.

T4 is required for the muscles of the stomach and intestines to push food along for digestion and excretion. When there isn't enough T4 present as in hypothyroidism, food absorption is slow, which can result in delayed bowel movements or constipation. This is different from hyperthyroidism, which usually results in diarrhea.

The heart plays a special role in metabolism. Thyroid hormone makes the heart beat faster, and when the heart beats faster, body temperature is raised. When the heart beats faster and body temperature is higher, the body increases the rate at which metabolism moves. The body doesn't have to be in motion to set internal signals of motion —if basal temperatures are warm and the heart beats at an accelerated rate, the body will need to use energy by burning calories. Because hypothyroid patients often feel cold and have slower heartbeats, their bodies metabolize fewer calories, which make weight loss seem like an impossible task.

Time for a heart to heart

Did you know that the less blood your heart pumps, the weaker it is? For women 55 and older, hypothyroidism is linked to heart attack risk (Annals of Internal Medicine, 2000; 132: 270-8). Low blood pressure can result in low energy and muscle wasting. In hypothyroid patients, the heart doesn't pump proper amounts of coronary circulation, which can result in heart failure. On the her hand, if the heart pump out more blood than it's ~~sed~~ to, the body feels as if it's running a nonstop ~~arathon~~, which can also lead to other problems like ~~adrenal~~ exhaustion.

In separate studies, Dr. Ahak (Ahak, A.E. et al. ~~hypothyroids and myocardial infractions"~~) and researchers at ~~Erasmus~~ University's medical school (D. Rotterdam. ~~Netherlands~~. *Annals of International Medicine*, 2000; 132: 270- ~~showed~~ hypothyroidism can cause myocardial ~~infarctions~~ in elderly women. Menopausal and post-~~menopausal~~ women who've been diagnosed with ~~hypothyroid~~ have a much greater likelihood of ~~developing~~ cardiovascular diseases than women who ~~have~~ a normal functioning thyroid. This is a scary stat, ~~especially~~ since we know that "20 percent of American ~~women~~ have been diagnosed with sub-clinical ~~hypothyroid~~." Although the data shows 20 percent, I'm ~~convinced~~ that this number is much, much higher.

Hyperthyroidism

Less common than hypothyroidism, ~~hyperthyroidism~~ is a condition that affects a few hundred ~~thousand~~ Americans each year and the consequences are ~~monstrous~~. Hyperthyroidism occurs when an overactive ~~thyroid~~ gland produces an excessive amount of thyroid ~~hormones~~ that circulate in the blood.

Hyperthyroid patients sweat more than ~~hypothyroid~~ patients because their bodies constantly ~~have~~ the heat on. The increased blood flow from an ~~increase~~ in thyroid hormone makes the hair greasy, the ~~hands~~ clammy, and the skin moist, wet and dewy.

In hypothyroid patients, the opposite occurs — ~~instead~~ of moist skin, they have dry skin, brittle nails, ~~and~~ fragile hair that falls out.

Gary's Story

Years ago while in med school, I clearly remember Gary, one of my classmates from a molecular biology course. He seemed so sharp; everything seemed to come easy to him. Any time the professor would ask a question that required contemplation or intense problem-solving, Gary would answer on the spot. He was a genius. At least he looked like he was studying more than any of the other classmates because he had the worst appearance. His eyelashes looked like they'd been glued to his eyebrows. He had these big, bulgy brown eyes with infinitesimal-looking red blood vessels, which seemed to congregate around the spherical border of both his pupils.

Gary agreed to help me study for the next exam. While we studied, I noticed he didn't drink coffee, yet he was so antsy. For such a skinny guy, Gary seemed to eat enormous amounts of food, all the time, around the clock. He confessed that he always had a hunger that couldn't be satisfied. Along with faint tremors, the inability to sit still, bulgy eyes and the desire to eat all the time, he took excessive amounts of bathroom breaks.

Gary suffered from a hyperactive thyroid. Patients with hyperthyroidism have such elevated sugar and accelerated basal metabolism that their bodies absorb food at an accelerated pace, which in turn creates a never-ending craving for sugar. This almost always leads to diabetes.

Testimonial

"Graduating college early at 20, I became a laboratory technician. Subconsciously, I think I have been competing with my boyfriend of three years who is an overachiever. He obtained his bachelor's in two years while teaching swimming lessons to 4-year-olds. Today, he is in law school, soon to graduate. I am still contemplating my next move. He motivates me to push myself, but I feel as if I have overdone it.

"Although I hadn't seen the doctor in months, I felt fairly certain that something was gravely wrong with me. I broke up with my boyfriend and made an appointment to see my physician after experiencing a series of mentally and emotionally paralyzing symptoms. As I sneezed my way into the doctor's office, I told her I had not yet recovered from a cold I had developed two months ago. Concerned about my overly active lifestyle and sickly condition, she conducted the works.

"After checking my temperature and advising me to check my own throughout the following day, I recalled my doctor holding her head while telling me exactly what the problem was--it was my thyroid. My doctor convinced me that complete recovery may not happen within a few days, but surely would within weeks.

"I was eager to begin treatment. The assessment made me realize how delicate the thyroid is, and that it can be triggered by an array of factors like stress, a lack of iodine and periods of dieting and self-starvation. I had done all of those things to myself, and as a result experienced painful PMS symptoms, cramps, dizzy spells and unending nausea.

"Thankfully, my doctor refused to aimlessly lure me into the world of pharmaceuticals. She had me take a natural iodine supplement and suggested I take up yoga or tai-chi. I did so. After nine hours in the lab, yoga seemed relieving and refreshing.

"My body reacted well to the iodine supplement I was prescribed, and because I followed instructions exactly as they were given to me, most of PMS symptoms have been alleviated and I feel less cold. I now leave my pullovers and knit-wear at home in the winter drawer where they belong."--Jasmine, 25

Low sex drive and the thyroid

Because the thyroid plays such a vital role in the body, the body enters a state of trauma when thyroid hormones are either overproduced or under produced.

Experiencing such burdening internal stressors can make you anxious, nervous and tense. These are all normal feelings (especially when you look in the mirror and are highly disappointed in the person you see). When weight-loss or weight-gain attempts have been unsuccessful, your hair falls out easily and your heart beats at an uncomfortable pace, it's no wonder the libido is affected. Besides sex being psychologically undesirable, sex will be physiologically undesirable as well for three reasons: your body is producing irregular amounts of T4 (and predictably T3); in women, menstruation cycles are skipped, thus stopping the production and ovulation of eggs; and the body experiences such a discomfort where it becomes confused as to how it should act, and so much confusion will result in an indifference towards pleasurable acts such as sex.

Thyroid dysfunction can impair a person's social life; they become too jittery for anyone to tolerate, or too fatigued to want to be social.

More serious conditions of the thyroid

GRAVES' DISEASE

Graves' disease is the most common form of hyperthyroidism. It occurs when a person's immune system mistakenly attacks their thyroid gland and causes it to overproduce the T4 hormone. The abnormal immune response can affect the tissue behind the eyes as well as parts of the skin. The higher the T4 level in Graves' disease can greatly increase your body's metabolic rate, leading to host of health problems.

Graves' disease is rarely life-threatening. Although it may develop at any age and in either men or women, Graves' disease is more common in women and usually begins after age 20.

There's no way to stop the immune system from attacking the thyroid gland, but treatments for Graves' disease can ease symptoms and decrease the production of thyroxine (T4).

HYPERTHYROID SYMPTOMS

- Heart palpitations
- Heat intolerance
- Nervousness
- Insomnia
- Breathlessness
- Increased bowel movements
- Light or absent menstrual periods
- Fatigue
- Fast heart beat
- Trembling hands
- Weight loss
- Muscle weakness
- Warm, moist skin
- Hair loss
- Staring gaze

HASHIMOTO'S THYROIDITIS

Hashimoto's thyroiditis, the most common cause of hypothyroidism in the United States, is a condition caused by inflammation of the thyroid gland. Since it is an autoimmune disease, the body inappropriately attacks the thyroid gland--as if it was foreign tissue. Hashimoto's thyroiditis tends to occur in families, and is associated with other autoimmune conditions such as Type 1 diabetes.

Hashimoto's thyroiditis is 5 to 10 times more common in women than in men and most often starts in adulthood. The symptoms of Hashimoto's thyroiditis are similar to those of hypothyroidism in general, which are often subtle.

The symptoms generally become more obvious as the condition worsens and the majority of these complaints are related to a metabolic slowing of the body.

Properly diagnosed, hypothyroidism can be easily and completely treated with thyroid hormone replacement. On the other hand, untreated hypothyroidism can lead to an enlarged heart (cardiomyopathy), worsening heart failure, and an accumulation of fluid around the lungs.

A man ahead of his time

During nearly 50 years of clinical practice, Dr. Broda Barnes, M.D., Ph.D., became an authority in the diagnosis and treatment of hypothyroidism. Seeing thousands of people suffering from undiagnosed cases of hypothyroidism led him to write a popular book called *"Hypothyroidism: The Unsuspected Illness"*.

It all started when he conducted an extensive analysis of the records of people who died in Graz, Austria during World War II. After reviewing records from the city's National Hospital, he found that after the war people began to die from infectious diseases. When antibiotics were finally administered, people then died from coronary artery diseases. This led him to make the correlation between infections and the heart, but "what," he thought, "what could trigger both?"

It wasn't until the mid-1970s when Dr. Barnes discovered the relationship between the two—it was the thyroid gland that was causing infections and deaths in these people.

Dr. Barnes noted that hypothyroidism often goes undiagnosed because blood thyroid values are usually inaccurate. Way ahead of his time, Dr. Barnes showed that an excellent indicator of the thyroid condition is basal body temperature, which the patient can perform at home.

How to perform the basal body temperature test

Dr. Barnes has found the basal temperature to be one of the most valid tests to evaluate thyroid function.

DIRECTIONS:

1) If you are male or a non-menstruating female, take an oral mercury thermometer (which has been shaken down and placed at the bedside the previous evening) and place it in your armpit for 10 minutes immediately upon awakening <u>while lying quietly in bed</u>. You must do this before getting up to do anything—even going to the bathroom. Repeat the test three days in a row. Normal temperature is 97.8 degrees to 98.2 degrees. If your temperature is low, your thyroid gland is probably underactive.

2) If you are a menstruating female, do the above test on the second and third day of your period in the same manner.

3) Record your results and take them to your physician.

DOES THIS SOUND LIKE YOU?

You may have a thyroid deficiency if you have:	You may have a thyroid excess if you have:
❑ Lethargy and decreased energy ❑ Intolerance to coldness ❑ Tingling and numbness in extremities ❑ Muscle pain and stiffness ❑ Constipation ❑ Weight gain ❑ Dry, scaly or yellowish skin ❑ Coarse hair and skin ❑ Depression ❑ Forgetfulness ❑ Personality changes ❑ Anemia ❑ Prolonged or heavy menstrual cycles	❑ Heart palpitations ❑ Heat intolerance ❑ Nervousness ❑ Insomnia ❑ Breathlessness ❑ Increased bowel movements ❑ Light or absent menstrual periods ❑ Fatigue ❑ Fast heart beat ❑ Trembling hands ❑ Weight loss ❑ Muscle weakness ❑ Warm, moist skin ❑ Hair loss ❑ Staring gaze
If you already use a thyroid support supplement, **increase** your dosage if the above symptoms are experienced.	If you already use a thyroid support supplement, **decrease** your dosage if the above symptoms are experienced.

ᘒ Dr. Tai's Amazing Beauty Secret ᘒ

As with any part of the body, the absolute best way to treat it is naturally. Remember, the thyroid is an extremely sensitive gland—too much will affect the way you feel, and too less of the thyroid hormone will also affect you, both in very negative ways. With the thyroid, you must be at a balance to feel yourself. It's a sensitive gland that can cause eye problems, breathing problems, and psychotic disorders and throw off your metabolism beyond the point of no return.

If you're experiencing minor thyroid symptoms, the worst thing you could do to yourself is pick up your doctor's prescription at the drug store. It's almost guaranteed that you will experience further problems in the future. However, if you're showing major signs of severe thyroid dysfunction, you'll have no choice but take extreme measures. Follow doctor's orders, but if you can avoid taking synthetic thyroid support, it would be wise to do so because many synthetic forms of thyroids are known for promoting brutal side effects such as weight gain, anaemia, elevated fats, disturbances in heart rhythm, convulsions, mild to severe forms of anxieties and so on.

Helpful hints for the thyroid...

- Take a supplement with selenium and iodine extracts from seaweed and seafood.
- Stay away from binge diets—no yo-yo dieting!! Do it the right way or don't do it all! Starving yourself will only hurt your thyroid and you'll accomplish only gaining back the pounds lost the previous month.
- Breathe deeply. Deep breathing exercises increases ATP Adenosine Triphosphate; ATP fuels the cells within our body with oxygen. ATP is the source of all your energy.
- To be sexy is to be comfortable. Don't attempt to sex up your image by wearing nearly nothing during cold months. Throwing basal temperatures off can "tinker with' de thyroid, man." If you're cold, put on a sweater!

Help your thyroid the natural way

- *Exercise moderately*
- *Eat foods rich in iodine*
- *Natural supplements of iodide/Iodine*
- *Natural thyroid supplements*

CHAPTER 21

Cortisol and Adrenaline: The stress hormones

"Stress is poison."

~Agavé Powers

If you are like most people, you occasionally find yourself hitting bumps in the road and getting stressed out over such things as money, kids, your job, or your spouse. As I'm sure you are well aware of, stress can really do a number on our looks and our health. If we want to look years younger, we need to make sure the stress in our lives is under control. Luckily, we have our adrenal glands, which act as shock absorbers for our body and determine our response to stress. Their role is to maintain and protect our health. Many body systems depend on these extraordinary glands for support, such as hormone balance, blood sugar control mechanisms, proper brain function, and proper function of the immune system.

These hard working glands regularly produce a variety of hormones for us such as:

- Cortisol to help us handle stress
- Hormones for emergencies, like adrenaline
- Melatonin for good sleep
- Various hormones to maintain our hydration

Adrenal Overview

The adrenals secrete catecholamine adrenaline (epinephrine), a hormone that pushes a person to react to stress. If it weren't for two hormones, adrenaline and cortisol, our bodies wouldn't know how to react in and recover from stressful situations. Cortisol and adrenaline are produced by the adrenal glands, the two pyramid-shaped structures that sit on top of the kidneys—one gland on each kidney.

Each of the adrenal glands has an outer part called the adrenal cortex and an inner part called the adrenal medulla.

Adrenal Cortex

Approximately 80 percent of an adrenal gland is its adrenal cortex. The adrenal cortex actually produces more than two-dozen steroid hormones called corticosteroids (kawr-tih-koh-STEER-oydz). One of these hormones is aldosterone (al-DAHS-tuh-rohn), a mineral hormone that prevents water retention by controlling the volume of sodium fluid in the body. Another hormone, called cortisol, helps control the metabolism rate of carbohydrates, fats, and proteins.

What does cortisol do?	
* Balances blood sugar	* Influences mood
* Helps weight control	* Affects testosterone/estrogen ratio
* Improves immune response	* Helps bone metabolism
* Affects DHEA/Insulin ratio	* Balances stress response

Adrenal Medulla

The sympathetic nervous system, which prepares the body for energy intense activities, regulates the release of hormones from the adrenal medulla. Two hormones released from the adrenal medulla are epinephrine (a.k.a adrenaline) and norepinephrine. Epinephrine, which is more powerful than norepinephrine, makes up about 80 percent of the total secretions of the adrenal medulla.

Adrenaline and noradrenalin are two hormones directly related to "fight or flight."

This response is the feeling you get when you are excited or frightened. Nerve impulses from the sympathetic nervous system stimulate cells and this stimulation causes the cells to release large amounts of epinephrine and norepinephrine. These hormones increase your heart rate, blood pressure, and blood flow to the muscles. They cause air passageways to open wider, allowing for an increase in oxygen intake. They also stimulate the release of extra glucose into the blood to help produce a sudden burst of energy. The result of all these actions is a general increase in body activity. If your heart rate speeds up and your hands begin to sweat when you get nervous, you are feeling the effects of your adrenal medulla!!

Adrenaline rush

As mentioned earlier, adrenaline is known as the "fight or flight" hormone, and plays a key role in the short-term stress reaction. When danger is present or during an emergency, adrenaline is released from the adrenal glands — hence referred to as an "adrenaline rush."

Adrenaline triggers may be threatening, exciting, or environmental stressor conditions such as high noise levels, or bright light, or extreme temperatures.

In the right amounts, adrenaline leaves you energized and makes you hyper, jumpy, happy and feeling a little crazy. But it's the good crazy, the kind that makes you feel like you can take on the world.

When epinephrine is released into the blood stream, it quickly prepares the body for action in emergency situations. In addition, the brain and muscles get a boost of oxygen and glucose, while other non-emergency bodily processes such as digestion are suppressed.

Adrenaline increases the heart rate and stroke volume, dilates the pupils, and contracts arterioles in the skin and gastrointestinal tract. In addition, the blood sugar level is increased while at the same time begins to breakdown lipids in fat cells. As with other stress hormones, epinephrine suppresses the immune system.

Cortisol, the regulator

The hormone cortisol is crucial to our survival. Produced under stress, cortisol is responsible for maintaining the ability to process sugars, sustain blood pressure and react to stress that can cause illness. As an adversary to insulin, cortisol breaks down carbohydrates and proteins; relieves inflammation, and allows the body to adapt to a broad range of circumstances. However, possessing a high cortisol level for an extended period of time leads to obesity, high blood pressure and adrenal fatigue. On the other hand, low cortisol levels can lead to chronic fatigue and stress-related disorders.

Elevated cortisol levels

Highly trained athletes generally possess higher-than-normal cortisol levels as well as women in the last trimester of pregnancy. Individuals suffering from depression, anxiety, panic disorder, malnutrition and alcohol abuse are also known to have elevated cortisol levels due to the increased physical and psychological stresses associated with these conditions.

What happens when cortisol is released?

- Muscle protein breaks down, leading to the release of amino acids into the bloodstream

- Gluconeogenesis then occurs as liver uses the amino acids to synthesize glucose for energy.

- This process raises the blood sugar level so the brain will have more glucose for energy. At the same time, other body tissues decrease their use of glucose as fuel.

- Cortisol also leads to the release of fatty acids, an energy source from fat cells, for use by the muscles.

- Together, these energy-directing processes prepare the individual to deal with stresses and ensure that the brain receives adequate energy supplies.

Almost immediately after a stressful event, the levels of the regulatory hormones adrenocorticotrophin (ACTH) and corticotrophin-releasing hormone (CRH) increase, causing an immediate rise in cortisol levels. Cortisol production, in amounts produced at the right time, helps heal tissues as well as protect the body by transporting available sugars for proper nutrition meant for healing. As a tissue builder, cortisol in minimal amounts can assist in retarding the aging process and fight fatigue.

What triggers abnormal cortisol levels?

Menopause	Panic disorder
Chronic fatigue syndrome	PMS
Fibromyalgia	Infertility
Depression	Sleep disorders
Impotence	Osteoporosis
Anorexia nervosa	Heart disease

(Heller, L., The essentials of Herbal Care Part II. Metagenics, Inc., 2000, p.1144)

Hard at work

Cortisols primary duty is attempting to make peace with invaders who use stress to attack and to impede excessive inflammation they may cause. These stressors can be physical, environmental, mental or emotional. An example of environmental stress would be if you're experiencing uncomfortable body temperatures, like being too hot or too cold. Another example is being in stressful environments where you are often exposed to loud noise, people who habitually argue in your presence, or it can even be working or living in a messy, unorganized or polluted environment.

From temperature to hygiene, various forms of stress provoke aggressive behavior — excess cortisol is released from your adrenal cortex. After enough cortisol production, glucose and glycogen (sugar) reserves are used to produce energy reactions (e.g., outbursts, verbal or physical gestures).

Symptom Checklist

If you are experiencing the following symptoms, you may be suffering from adrenal overload or exhaustion.

- fatigue (often a pattern of morning or evening fatigue)
- insomnia
- fatigue after intense exercise
- worsened signs of hormone imbalance or trouble getting hormones balanced
- trouble focusing or poor memory
- anxiety
- depression
- cravings, especially for sweets or carbs
- low blood sugar symptoms
- weight gain, especially around the middle

Adrenal burnout!!

Beware! Release of too much cortisol can and will burn out the adrenals. If you are one who is always on the go and always stressed out, be careful! Exhausted adrenals cause people to biologically age sooner by suppressing their immune systems and thinning their skin. Excessive cortisol production will eventually cause deep lines and wrinkles.

Within our society, people are confronted with all sorts of obstacles they are expected to overcome. As a result, our bodies have become accustomed to producing more and more cortisol. In fact, many people function solely on cortisol. Besides toothpicks, cortisol seems to be the only thing that keeps people's eyes open during the day. Cortisol is continuously released when we don't get enough sleep. Since so much of the hormone is used up on a daily basis, the body uses up cortisol reserves, causing depletion to occur much sooner than expected. Then.... adrenal fatigue sets in.

When constant demand is placed on the adrenals, they become tired and "exhausted." Someone with adrenal exhaustion may: feel stressed out, have a short temper, lack focus, and have low energy levels. The increased production of adrenal hormones which occurs with stress increases the metabolism of protein, fats, carbohydrates, therefore producing instant energy for the body to use. But as more stress is placed on the adrenals, the weaker they become. When this happens, our body reacts negatively and conditions such as ulcers, hypertension, backaches, allergies, infections, weakened immune system, weight gain, lack of energy, and insomnia often develop.

Cortisol and weight gain

Did you know?

If you are trying to lose weight, it doesn't help matters much just sitting behind your desk stressing out. Because our body is not using the extra sugar energy (produced by stress) to fight off or run away from some "man-eating" animal, the excess sugar with no place to go turns into fat cells as stored energy. These fat cells then accumulate around our waist and all over our body, making us fat and eventually obese.

- Excess cortisol levels increase fat deposits around waist and abdomen.
- Increased cortisol values also increase the chances of early memory loss, hypertension and cardiovascular disease.

When you feel stressed and tired, don't try fighting the fatigue. Give in for once! If you feel tired, try some deep breathing exercises, close your eyes for a few minutes or splash some cold water on the back of your neck and wrists. Do something to calm down during moments of stress. Remember, short-term stressors can have very negative long-term effects. It's your body telling you it needs rest, quiet repair and sleep.

Athletes and workaholics

What do athletes and workaholics have in common? They both have higher than normal cortisol levels that will only cause problems for them.

Like athletes, workaholics are all about achieving their goals in an all-or-nothing way. They savor their workload, they're relentless, and they have trouble stopping what they're doing only to make careless mistakes along the way, which end up working against them. Obsessing over details to the point of paralysis, perfectionists and overachievers have what I like to call a "hero complex." They get kudos from their professional superiors and they give the impression that they are capable of things above and beyond the call of duty. They're slaves in their own offices, attached to their desks or, in an athlete's case, the gym, track, court or field. This can be because they try to avoid going home, or maybe don't have much of a social life. As

ith everything, cases vary and everything is relative, but one thing remains absolute —
orkaholics and athletes have higher than normal cortisol levels that will only lead to their
emise amidst what could become potential glory.

he over-trained athlete

After researching
ntrained and trained athletes
nd athletes who are over-
rained, I can certainly see a
imilar pattern in our over-
rained athletes who have
drenal fatigue, and therefore
heir cortisol hormone levels are
ery low as a response to their
raining activities.

Losing the Game

Recovery periods for athletes typically last around 48 hours. If athletes don't allow sufficient time for their muscles to repair after an intense workout, the body's immune system is sure to be weakened. During the 48-hour healing period, DHEA and cortisol are released in the blood as a mending mechanism for damaged tissues. At the end of this period, cortisol slows in production to relieve the body of feeling overwhelmed or over-burdened, replenishing and preparing the body for additional activity.

Die-hard athletes are more susceptible to allergies, colds and injuries, more so than people who exercise reasonably. This is why it's especially important for athletes to take a day or two off after intense training to allow their bodies to repair muscles and foster immunities. By not allowing their muscles sufficient time to recover, athletes risk permanent injury in which recovery is not possible. Overtraining, not under-training is the athlete's worst enemy.

Low cortisol levels cause these athletes to have much more inflammatory reaction,
muscle protein and tissue breakdown, more pain and discomfort post-training, and delayed
healing and recovery time. These fatigued, over-trained athletes require greater rest and more
ime to recuperate and heal from their training. Pushing and going back to training before the
ody is ready will only exacerbate and make their already broken tissues even worse,
ultimately causing permanent damage or injury from which they are unable to recover.

DOES THIS SOUND LIKE YOU?

You may have a cortisol deficiency if you have:	You may have a cortisol excess if you have:
❑ Insomnia ❑ Fatigue ❑ Digestive problems ❑ Emotional imbalances ❑ Loss of sexual interest ❑ Low blood pressure ❑ Low blood sugar ❑ Slow heartbeat ❑ Severe fatigue ❑ Sugar craving ❑ Stressed ❑ Light headed from sitting or standing	❑ Sleep problems ❑ Sugar cravings ❑ Memory problems ❑ Osteoporosis ❑ Lack of energy ❑ High blood pressure ❑ High cholesterol & triglyceride levels ❑ Water retention ❑ Elevated blood sugar ❑ Thinning skin ❑ Loss of muscle mass ❑ Anxiety, irritability and nervousness ❑ Feelings of stress ❑ Weight gain—especially around the middle ❑ Arthritis and muscle pain ❑ Hair loss
If you already use an adrenal support supplement, **increase** your dosage if the above symptoms are experienced.	If you already use an adrenal support supplement, **decrease** your dosage if the above symptoms are experienced.

José's Story

"Ever since I was a young child, my role models have always been athletes. My dad, an immigrant from Mexico, was a phenomenal athlete, but he never had the opportunity to pursue his interests in football because he had to work to support his family. While other kids climbed trees and built forts, I ran. In fact, running is all I've ever done.

At 5-foot-10, coaches were constantly telling me that I was built to run—strong legs, upright and aligned posture with long, lean arms. I had enough muscle strength to carry me through the nastiest weather conditions and roughest terrain. Whether it be high winds, traffic, pounding rain or a snow blizzard, I made sure to get an early-morning run before school and a late-evening run after working or studying. My dad encouraged me to train more instead of working for our family business because he knew how much running meant to me. So I did and I devoted my senior year to burning out my adrenals.

As a high-school senior, different universities were looking to recruit students for their team. And I had my heart set on Syracuse University. I wanted nothing more than a full-ride scholarship to a highly regarded school like Syracuse. I planned ongoing pre-med and to be known as campus' Jersey boy who shattered records."

But I made the mistake of over-training. I trained to the point of exhaustion. My daily routine consisted of back strengthening, bicep curls, chest strengthening, leg strengthening, curls, shoulder presses, a five-mile morning run and a three-mile evening run.

In March, I developed a deadly cold which I couldn't recover from. As soon as I thought I was better, I got worse. Finally, when Syracuse came to visit the school, they weren't impressed by me. My performance was horrendous and I had made running look painful. I blew my chances of making the team because I over-trained. It took my body months to recover from exhaustion and depression. I was really hard on myself. In the end, I got accepted to Syracuse, but not on a sports scholarship.

I'm currently a junior at Syracuse and I've learned not to be so hard on myself. It was unfortunate that I had to learn the hard way. This year, I'm taking it easy. I'm worrying about my G.P.A. and only training lightly. If I make the track team when the season arrives, I make the team—if I don't, then that too will be OK. Right now, my health is my top priority."

~José, 22

❧ DR. TAI'S AMAZING BEAUTY SECRET ❧

As I've said time after time, health and appearance are related to each other. The adrenal glands play an important role in producing a variety of hormones, specifically cortisol. However, cortisol production is like a double-edged sword. If the body doesn't produce enough cortisol, a person isn't as alert as they should be. But if the body produces too much cortisol, a person's chances of turning into a worn-out sugar junkie greatly increases.

Excess cortisol levels can lead to dementia, insomnia and obesity because the hormone acts as a metabolic inhibitor, affecting the receptors in the body by pushing sugar to deposit into fat at great speeds. Invariably, this affects your appearance, causing weight to congregate at the waist, as in apple-shaped bodies (wide hips and thin legs).

Even if you only vaguely suspect you may an adrenal hormone excess, I highly recommend you get your saliva tested. The slightest amount of an adrenal hormone excess can throw a person off balance, placing them into a never ending lose-lose situation, where for a short time the rush is felt but is then paid for in the long run.

Through saliva testing, people who lead active or stressful lifestyles can be helped by evaluating their biomarkers. Hormones mark how much energy a person possesses and how healthy the person is. By measuring saliva, we can evaluate cortisol, testosterone and DHEA and help people maximize their energy potential.

By making the right lifestyle choices such as dieting, bioidentical hormone replacement and moderate exercise, you'll be able to avoid the mental and emotional havoc that excess cortisol produces.

RESOURCES

Health Secrets USA
24141 Ann Arbor Trail
Dearborn Heights MI 48127
Tel: 313.561.6800
Fax: 313.561.6830
info@healthsecretsusa.com
Website: http://www.healthsecretsusa.com

Get Healthy Again
Robert Harrison
40374 Waterman Road
Homer AK 99603
Tel: 907-235-5556
Website: http://www.gethealthyagain.com

Healthy Get Items
PO Box 2308
Birmingham MI 48012
Website: http://www.healthygetitems.com

REFERENCES

A

Since 1997, there has been a 457 percent increase in the total number of cosmetic procedures. Surgical procedures increased by 114 percent, and nonsurgical procedures increased by 754 percent.

*According to the American Society for Aesthetic Plastic Surgery

* Premarin made from horse's estrogens, equilin and equilenin can cause side effects such as burning on urination, allergies, joint aches, and pains.

Ahlgrimm, M., The HRT Solution. 1999; New York: Avery Pub.

Estrogens derived from horses urine may stay in your body up to 13 weeks, in contrast to your natural estradiol which are eliminated from your body within a few hours.

Ahlgrimm, M., The HRT Solution. 1999; New York: Avery Pub.

What can DHEA do?

(Ahlgrimm, M., The HRT Solution 1999; New York: Avery Pub.)

Hypothyroidism is an indicator of atherosclerosis and myocardial infarction in elderly women (Annals of Internal Medicine, 2000; 132: 270-8).

(Ahak, A.E. et al. "Hypothyroids and myocardial infractions") and researchers at Erasmus University's medical school (D. Rotterdam. Netherlands. *Annals of International Medicine,* 2000; 132: 270-8.

High levels of DHEA may retard the development of coronary atherosclerosis and coronary vasculopathy. (*Annals of New York Academy of Sciences,* December, 1995; 774:271-80.)

B

Bland J., "Obesity and endocrine signaling." Health Comm International, Inc. 1999, p.124.

(Baulieu, E.E., et al. "DHEA Sulfate and aging contribution of the DHEA age study to socio-biomedical." *Proceedings from the National Academy of Sciences USA,* 2000; 97(8)4279-4284).

C

(Collins, J., What's Your Menopause Type. Roseville, CA: Prima Health 2000).

E

(Erskin et al. "Iodine response in rates." *Biological Trace Element Research, 1995; 49;209-219.)*

F

(Flood, J. F., et al. "Memory-enhancing effects in male mice of pregnenolone and steroids metabolically derived from it." *Proceedings from the National Academy of Science of the United State of America,* 1992; 89:1567-71).

(Freeman, H., et al. "Therapeutic efficacy of pregnenolone in rheumatoid arthritis." *The Journal of the American Medical Association,* 1950; 143: 338-44.)

H

"Obesity and endocrine signaling." Health Comm International, Inc. 1999, p.124.)

J

In men, there was a small rise of androstenedione. Perceived physical and psychological well-being rose by 67 percent in men and 84 percent in women. (*Journal of Clinical Endocrinology and Metabolism,* June 1994; 78(6): 1360)

High levels of DHEA inhibit the development of atherosclerosis.(*Journal of Clinical Investigations,* August, 1998; 82(2): 712-20)

HGH decreases by 75 percent from adulthood to midlife. HGH loss is complete by age 40. (*The Journal of the American Medical Association,* August, 2000; 284(7): 861-866.)

In order to maintain optimal brain function, older patients may require middle to high level circulating thyroid. Hypothyroid patients may suffer subtle cognitive deficits. (*Journal of Gerontology: Medical Sciences,* 1999; 54A (3): M111-M116)

(Women's Health Initiative research team. "Risks and benefits of estrogen and progesterone in healthy post-menopausal women." *Journal of the American Medical Association,* 2002; 288:321-333.)

K

Low dose growth hormone treatment with diet restriction accelerates body fat loss, exerts anabolic effect and improves growth hormone secretory dysfunction in obese adults.   Kim KR, et al. Horm Res 1999; 511(2) :78-8.

L

DHEA Benefits (Lieberman, S., The Real Vitamin and Mineral Book. NY: Avery Pub. 1997)

(Labrie, C. and Belanger, A., et al. "High bioavailability of DHEA administered percutaneously in the rat." Journal of Endocrinology, 1996; 150: S107-118.)

(Lee, J.R., What Your Doctor May Not Tell You About Menopause. Warner Books, May, 1996).

(Lee, J.R. "Osteoporosis reversal with transdermal progesterone." Lancet, 1990; 336:1327.)

The Power of Natural Progesterone (Laux, M., Natural Woman, Natural Menopause, NY:HarperCollins, 1997)

(Lieberman, S., The Real Vitamin and Mineral Book. Avery Publ. 1997,.p.216

M

(McCormick, D. L. and Rao, K.V.N., et al. "Chemoprevention of hormone dependent prostate cancer in wistar unilever rats." The Journal of European Urology, 1999; 35: 464-467.)

(McGavack, T., et al. "The use of pregnenolone in various clinical disorders." Journal of Clinical Endocrinology and Metabolism, 1951; 11: 559-77.)

N

(Baulieu, E.E., et al. "DHEA Sulfate and aging contribution of the DHEA age study to socio-biomedical." Proceedings from the National Academy of Sciences USA, 2000; 97(8)4279-4284).

HGH improves quality of life, including: energy level, mood and emotions. (New England Journal of Medicine, October 1999; 341:1206-1216.)

P

Because ovaries have thyroid receptors and the thyroid gland has ovarian receptors, losing testosterone and Estradiol during menopause can cause lower thyroid function and production. (Pamela, S. HRT, The Answers. Healthy Living Books. 2003)

S

(Schwartz, Arthur. "Cancer prevention with DHEA." *Journal of Cellular Biochemistry*, 1995; 59(S22):210-217.)

Synthetic Estrogen is not compatible to your body's estrogen receptors. *Sinatra, S., Heart Sense for Women. Washington DC; Lifeline Press, 2000.*

Selye, H., et al. "Potentiation of a pituitary extract with pregnenolone and additional observations concerning the influence of various organs on steroids, metabolism." *Pineal Journal Review,* 1943; 10(2):319-28.)

Synthetic Estrogen is not compatible to your body's estrogen receptors. *Sinatra, S., Heart Sense for Women. Washington DC; Lifeline Press, 2000*

Y

A diet consisting of too much saturated fat and trans-fatty acids interferes and blocks with the natural pathway of pregnenolone. (*Yanick, P., Prohormone Nutrition, Montclair, NJ:Longevity Institute International, 1998.*)

INDEX